THE PSYCHOLOGICAL AND MEDICAL EFFECTS
OF CONCENTRATION CAMPS AND RELATED PERSECUTIONS
ON SURVIVORS OF THE HOLOCAUST

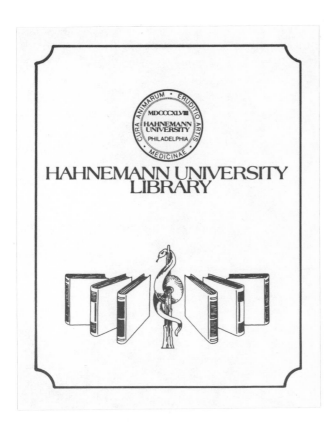

The Psychological and Medical Effects of Concentration Camps and Related Persecutions on Survivors of the Holocaust

A RESEARCH BIBLIOGRAPHY

by
Leo Eitinger
and
Robert Krell

with Miriam Rieck

University of British Columbia Press
Vancouver
1985

The Psychological and Medical Effects of Concentration Camps and Related
Persecutions on Survivors of the Holocaust: A Research Bibliography

© The University of British Columbia Press 1985

Canadian Cataloguing in Publication Data

Eitinger, Leo, 1912–
Psychological and medical effects of
concentration camps and related persecutions on survivors of the holocaust

Includes index.
ISBN 0-7748-0220-0

1. Holocaust, Jewish (1939– 1945) –
Psychological aspects – Bibliography.
2. Holocaust, Jewish (1939– 1945) –
Physiological aspects – Bibliography.
3. Holocaust survivors – Bibliography.
I. Krell, Robert. II. Title.
Z6374.H6E397 1985   016.94053'15'03924   C85-091346-2

International Standard Book Number 0-7748-0220-0

Printed in Canada

In Memory of the Victims
of the Holocaust

CONTENTS

FOREWORD

Recently there has been a growing worldwide interest in the various aspects of the Holocaust and its implications. While obviously important in its own right, it may well signify the gradually increasing detachment from that unique horror. Many scholars who only yesterday found it impossible to study a theme of such high personal involvement are finding it less and less difficult. No longer personally painful, yet not entirely distant, the Holocaust experience is situated in that grey no-man's-land which makes it for the first time in many years accessible to the objective investigation and mind. However, this may turn out to be short-lived interest, just as the candle, before dying out, flickers intensely just one more time.

The implications are clear. The concerned and responsible investigators cannot take any chances and must proceed with their work now, while it is still possible to do so. The survivors, that uniquely tragic breed, are dying out very fast and soon not a single one will be left. The research efforts concerning them should therefore be concentrated and carried out without delay.

In view of the importance of serious research, combined with its urgency and the difficulty in obtaining the available information which is dispersed all over the world, the Ray D. Wolfe Centre for Study of Psychological Stress was fortunate to have Professor Eitinger undertake the task of collecting all available material for a research bibliography. He is clearly among the best qualified in the world to contribute his broad scope and wisdom to this relatively neglected theme. During his stay with us, he not only initiated, carried through, and brought to successful completion the mammoth task of collecting material to provide a comprehensive volume, but at the same time raised the interests of many others, including Dr. Krell of the University of British Columbia, to complete and continue this work.

A research bibliography, in order to be effective, must be a living thing.

Even as this volume goes into print, numerous new studies are being carried out which ought to appear in subsequent editions. The bibliographical collection must be continuously updated and readily available to interested scholars. Our centre views the function of promoting research and information in this area not only its duty but a great honour. Anyone interested in reading and studying the research publications in their entirety is invited to come and use our special library. Too much has happened to too many for mankind ever to be satisfied with its understanding of the Holocaust.

Shlomo Breznitz
Lady Davis Professor
Director of the Ray D. Wolfe Centre for
Study of Psychological Stress.
University of Haifa

PREFACE

This research bibliography is the result of a collaborative effort. Hence, the preface reflects credit to those who assisted Professor Leo Eitinger and Miriam Rieck at the Ray D. Wolfe Centre for the Study of Psychological Stress at the University of Haifa, and those who assisted Dr. Robert Krell at the University of British Columbia, Vancouver, Canada.

In collecting, classifying, and computerizing the materials contained in this book, we have been helped by many people and institutions. We want to thank our colleagues from all over the world for sending us their papers and books which now form a comprehensive collection at three centres: The Ray D. Wolfe Centre for Study of Psychological Stress at the University of Haifa, and the Department of Psychiatry Library at the University of British Columbia, Vancouver, B.C., Canada, and more recently, Stichting ICODO in Utrecht, Holland.

In Haifa, we wish to thank the Strochlitz Foundation and Professor Vago, Head of the Chair of Holocaust Studies, who made possible the beginning of this work. It was mainly owing to Professor S. Breznitz, Director of the Ray D. Wolfe Centre for Study of Psychological Stress, his secretary, Mrs. R. Maoz, and all other members of the centre, that the initial bibliography was printed in booklet form. Mrs. Iris Fry and Mrs. Liora Komornic prepared the material for the computer; Mr. E. Adler, principal librarian for planning and development, computerized the list, aided by Mrs. Yehudith Yarkoni. Mrs. N. Abkin, head at the department for publication, prepared the material for print, and Mrs. J. Ben-Josef designed the cover for that booklet.

In Vancouver, we were helped by the U.B.C. Department of Psychiatry librarians, Mrs. Vinetta Lunn and Mr. Cliff Cornish, by Ms. Maureen Phillips (secretary), Ms. Colleen McEachern and Ms. Sheryl Davis (volunteers). While on leave in Los Angeles, one editor (R.K.) received generous assistance from the staff of the Simon Wiesenthal Center including Mrs. Marlene Hier, Dr. Alex Grobman, Rabbi Daniel

Landes, and Shera Cohn (secretary). A grant donated by Isadore and Sophie Waldman of Vancouver, B.C., assisted in many facets of production. Ms. Linda Dayan graciously designed the cover of this book. A special thanks to my wife, Marilyn Krell, and my children for their patience with my preoccupations.

Institutions which have directly or indirectly supported and encouraged our work include: The United States Holocaust Memorial Council, Washington, D.C.; The Norwegian Federation of War Disabled; The United States Veterans Administration; the University of Oslo; ICODO in Utrecht, Holland; the Canadian Jewish Congress, and the University of British Columbia.

Leo Eitinger, M.D.
Robert Krell, M.D.
Miriam Rieck, M.A.
(Research Assistant)

INTRODUCTION

Professor Eitinger and Miriam Rieck compiled a booklet of references in Haifa while Dr. Robert Krell was individually engaged in compiling a bibliography. Rather than produce two similar, perhaps incomplete works, it was decided in 1981 to produce one book.

In this book the reader will find a bibliographical list of studies of the medical and psychological sequelae of concentration camp incarceration and related persecutions published to 1984. The material was gathered from all over the world and represents practically all that has been written on the topic to the date of publication. And yet it is entirely possible that this collection is missing someone's work. If so, do not hesitate to send reprints or unpublished manuscripts for inclusion in a future edition.

The lists of this collection are computerized at both centres and will be continuously updated. A library of reprints and manuscripts exists at the University of Haifa where they can be seen and used. A similar collection is in formation at the University of British Columbia, and another at Stichting ICODO. Copies of papers can be provided on request from either the University of Haifa or the University of British Columbia, Department of Psychiatry library. A researcher interested in the medical and psychological consequences of concentration camp imprisonment and survivorhood can utilize one of these collections for his or her work.

There is a great amount of literature in many languages. The medical and psychiatric damage of incarceration is well documented. The remarkable adjustments by many survivors are not. This bibliography reflects the obvious slant towards individuals examined for psychological and medical difficulties, hence the emphasis on psychopathology.

From the recent literature, particularly in doctoral dissertations where control groups are used, a more equitable picture emerges between the adapted afflicted and maladapted afflicted, especially with respect to the consequences for children of survivors.

There is no doubt that this body of literature reflects the tragic and longlasting effects of the most pervasive trauma imaginable. It is an area deserving of further study, and it is hoped that the bibliography will assist students of the subject.

HOW TO USE THIS BIBLIOGRAPHY

The references cited are in many languages. In order to simplify matters somewhat, we chose to capitalize all words in German and Polish titles and to italicize the English translation to assist the reader visually.

The numbering system skips in increments of 10 from 00050 to 00060 etc. This system provides some latitude for the inclusion of late "finds" or last minute manuscripts submitted. Therefore, not all references will be designated with a "round" number but all references will *retain* the designated number. For example, 00960 will identify an author and the article and will remain so in the subject index. Where an author has contributed many articles over the years, e.g., Eitinger, they are listed in chronological sequence according to the date of publication.

The articles are drawn from the medical, psychological, psychiatric, and social work literature. A few may be considered marginally related, but they are included if the central theme contributes to the knowledge of "psychologic" consequences. The editors have chosen not to provide editorial comment by excluding articles, rather they have been over-inclusive. It is for the researcher who uses these materials to examine their worth critically.

The major topics fall into several identifiable categories but with considerable overlap. The following is a brief survey to familiarize the reader/researcher with the major topics. These broad-based topics are additionally categorized within the subject index.

A BRIEF SURVEY OF THE MAJOR TOPICS

I *Direct observation of, and direct reactions to the concentration camp during imprisonment and immediately after liberation.*

Papers and books in this category include personal descriptions of life in the concentration camp and a few reports on the state of the survivors immediately after liberation. At the time of liberation, little detailed research was done. Probably no one had expected such longlasting effects subsequent to concentration camp imprisonment. The degrees of trauma and torture had never before been encountered or described in the medical literature. There is a considerable time lapse between the appearance of the relatively few papers belonging to this category and the prolific literature emerging in the fifties and which continues to the present time.

It is worth noting that a number of medical observers commented on the need for massive psychologic rehabilitation to parallel the massive psychologic traumas sustained. Effective psychiatric intervention was limited by the overriding preoccupations with feeding the undernourished, sheltering the homeless, and reuniting fragments of families.

In the immediate post-war period, social agencies bore the brunt of front-line intervention. Psychologists and psychiatrists did not become directly involved with the emotional effects of the prolonged persecution until the refugees had found a homeland. Hence the sparse literature between 1945–50. In the fifties, the increase in the psychiatric literature is attributable to several factors. The survivors' immediate preoccupation with finding family, settling into a new homeland, and learning new languages gave way to despair. For some, their experiences caught up and overwhelmed them. In addition, survivors were being examined psychiatrically for compensation and therefore came to the attention of the mental health professions.

II *Compensation-Rehabilitation*

Survivors seeking compensation brought into focus the inadequacy of existing compensation laws. In the federal republic of Germany, these laws were based on the prevailing theories in German psychiatry. The major psychoses were considered endogenous and based on genetic predisposition, neuroses were caused by personality characteristics, while traumatic neuroses were considered as caused by a desire for compensation. Even those who accepted a modern and psychodynamic view could rely only on the psychoanalytic theory in respect to the genesis of the neuroses, requiring the antecedents of childhood experiences and traumatizations. Karl Jaspers' theory of psychogenic psychosis after a traumatic life event was also unable to explain the longlasting psychological disturbances. According to Jaspers, both the content of the psychosis and its duration after the trauma were closely related to it. There was no explanation for any post-traumatic chronic psychic disturbances.

It was thus difficult to convince the judges of the existence of a causal relationship between concentration camp experiences and the concentration camp survivor syndrome. The longlasting symptoms appearing after a latent period could not be related to an existing psychiatric theory. It was difficult to convince not only the judges but also those psychiatrists who served as experts in assisting the judges.

This state of affairs caused much additional suffering to survivors who only reluctantly and with great effort overcame their inhibition to again expose this part of their lives in order to ask the Germans for compensation. As a result of studies such as those done in Norway, the diseases of survivors in several countries are ascribed to their war experiences, unless the authorities can prove otherwise.

Compensation remains a contemporary issue for those who survived the war as children and who have suffered a breakdown in functioning many years after the event.

III *Physical and Psychological Results*

In the fifties, French, Danish, Dutch, and Polish authors reported mainly on the longlasting physical damage to survivors, though some references to psychic effects were made. A survey of this literature demonstrates general agreement among authors about the longlasting effects of starvation, infectious diseases, torture, and massive trauma. The clinical findings of longlasting somatic damage were corroborated in a well-controlled epidemiological study in Norway. The emphasis on somatic findings remains characteristic of the literature from eastern European countries during the sixties and the seventies, including reports on the second generation. This is in marked contrast to the literature emphasizing the psychologic sequelae which appeared in western Europe, North America, and Israel.

These papers with a distinct psychiatric focus appeared in the fifties and sixties. The most conspicuous feature of this subject is the unexpected clinical picture encountered by most authors. Contrary to what would have been predicted by the prevailing psychiatric and psychological theories, it was shown that:

1) The psychologic disturbances did not necessarily appear immediately after the trauma, but after the "latency or symptom-free period."
2) The symptoms did not subside in time. On the contrary, many became more accentuated over the years.
3) The proportion of survivors afflicted with psychic disturbances was very high.
4) Although the clinical picture was quite uniform among survivors, this picture did not fit any known psychological or psychiatric classification. The constellation of somatic and psychiatric symptoms became known as the "concentration camp or survivor syndrome."
5) Survivors did not respond well to classical psychotherapy. Psychotherapists encountered difficulties with their own need to deny the horrors undergone by their patients. Some relief was obtained for some patients by longlasting supportive therapy.

Much of this evidence is based on clinical impressions from work with survivors who sought psychotherapy, and therefore the findings were viewed as biased and not representative of all survivors. Whereas the lack of controlled studies cannot be ignored, the results obtained from well-controlled psychometric and psychodiagnostic tests must also be taken into account. The few studies that employ these methods do lend support to the clinical impressions.

IV *Children as Survivors*

This is an especially tragic chapter within the framework of this catastrophic event. It renders everyone who deals with the subject "less scientific" and personally vulnerable. Perhaps this explains partly the comparative sparsity of literature on this subject.

The proportion of children who are survivors of hiding is far greater than the number who survived concentration camps. Clear effects of persecution and war experiences for child survivors of camps, those in hiding or wandering, are complicated by the nature of the immediate postwar experience.

The consequences of the trauma endured were affected by such variables as reunion with one or both parents, adoption, foster homes and orphanages, Kibbutz placement, etc. Of these children, only a very few have been followed up in a systematic manner and relatively little is known of their adaptation.

V Second Generation

These papers first appeared in the sixties and were primarily based on clinical studies. Later material includes dissertations on nonclinical populations with control studies.

Conclusions drawn from this literature are not at all uniform but allow some generalized observations. Difficulties generally did not emerge until the children of survivors had reached adolescence. The difficulties seemed related to issues of separation and individuation, and it was assumed that the methods of child-rearing experienced did not properly prepare them for the normal process of disengagement from parental protection. However, there have been no studies that have interviewed survivors about their child-rearing practices, and it is not known that it is precisely these experiences which caused the problems.

Not infrequently, the atmosphere at home was influenced by the parental experiences and memories, with physical and financial security a major preoccupation. Second generation persons in need of care sometimes complain of having been told too much and therefore living in the shadow of the Holocaust; others of having been told too little, yet being similarly burdened.

A considerable amount of literature has emerged about the silent majority to whom these generalizations do not apply. Again, the problem of uncontrolled studies is in evidence as well as the fact that much work draws on a biased sample, those who actually present for psychiatric care. There remains a need for well-controlled scientific work to examine the effects of massive traumatization on subsequent generations.

Summary

As in other fields, findings were reviewed from time to time and the theoretical implications examined. The inadequacy of prevailing psychiatric and psychological theories in accounting for the sequelae to massive trauma was stressed, but no sound and comprehensive alternative theory has yet been presented.

The aforementioned topic areas or themes are very broad and in order to assist researchers, this bibliography offers a more specific subject index. For example, the somatic results can now be found under conditions pertaining to famine, typhus, tuberculosis, etc., and under body systems including cardiovascular, respiratory, dermatological and neurological symptomatology.

There is considerable overlap, since the various sequelae could be listed in some instances under immediate consequences and sometimes under late effects of the concentration camp experience.

We have taken our cue from key words in the title or from personal knowledge of an article's content. Numerous articles and books were put at our disposal by various authors in addition to personal communication with many. We have tried to include all known work and again invite you to apprise us of references to be included in the future. Copies of your work will be gratefully received and added to the reference libraries at the University of Haifa and the University of British Columbia.

THE BIBLIOGRAPHY

00050 ABEL, T.
The Sociology of Concentration Camps. Soc Forces (1951) 30:150–155.

00060 ADAMCZYK, A.
[*The Last Days in the Hospital of the Leitmeritz Camp*]. Przeglad
Lekarski (1980) 37(1):184–186.

00070 ADELSBERGER, L.
Auschwitz, Ein Tatsachenbericht. [*Auschwitz, A Factual Account*].
Berlin: Letner, 1956.

00080 ADELSBERGER, L.
Psychologische Beobachtungen Im Konzentrationslager Auschwitz.
[*Psychological Observations in the Concentration Camp Auschwitz*].
Psychol Schw Zschr F Psychol (1974) 6:124–131.

00090 ADELSON, D.
Some Aspects of Value Conflict under Extreme Stress. Psychiatry (1962)
25:273–279.

00100 ADLER, H.G.; LANGBEIN, H.; LINGENS, E.
Auschwitz, Zeugnisse, und Berichte. [*Auschwitz, Testimony and
Report*]. Frankfurt: Europaische Verlagsanstalt, 1962.

00110 ALEKSANDROWICZ, D.R.
Children of Concentration Camp Survivors. In Anthony, E.J., and
C. Koupernik, (eds.), The Child in His Family: The Impact of Disease
and Death. New York: Wiley, 1973, 385–392.

00120 ALEXANDER, L.
*Sociopsychologic Structure of the S.S.: Psychiatric Report of the
Nurnberg Trials for War Crimes.* Arch Neurol Psychiat (1948)
59:622–634.

00130 ALEXANDER, L.
War Crimes. Their Social-Psychological Aspects. Am J Psychiat (1948)
105:170–177.

00140 ALEXANDER, L.
Medical Science under Dictatorship. New Engl J Med (1949)
241(2):39–47.

00150 AMELUNXEN, U.
Herabsetzung Der Altersgrenzen In Der Sozialversicherung Für
Verfolgte Des National Sozialismus. [*Lowering the Age Limit in Social
Insurance for People Persecuted by the National Socialists*]. In Herberg,
H.J. (ed.), Spätschäden Nach Extrembelastungen. II Internationalen
Medizinisch-Juristischen Konferenz In Düsseldorf (1969). Herford:
Nicholaische Verlags Buchhandlung, 1971, 99–103.

00160 ANTHONY, E.J.
Symposium: *Children of the Holocaust*. Editorial Comment. In
Anthony, E.J., and C. Koupernik (eds.), The Child in His Family: The
Impact of Disease and Death. New York: Wiley, 1973, 352–356.

00170 ANTONOVSKY, A.; MAOZ, B.; DOWTY, N.; WIJSENBEEK, H.
*Twenty-Five Years Later: A Limited Study of Sequelae of the
Concentration Camp Experience*. Soc Psychiat (1971) 6(4):186–193.

00180 APOSTOL-STANISZEWSKA, J.
[*Reminiscences from the Brzezinka Concentration Camp for Women*].
Przeglad Lekarski (1977) 34(1):200–207.

00190 APOSTOL-STANISZEWSKA, J.
[*Facing Death at the Birkenau and Ravensbruck Concentration Camps*].
Przeglad Lekarski (1981) 38(1):163–168.

00200 APPELBERG, E.
Holocaust Survivors and Their Children. In Linzer, N., The Jewish
Family. New York: Commission on Synagogue Relations, Federation
of Jewish Philanthropies, 1972, 109–122.

00210 ARIETI, S.
The Prerequisites of Nazi Barbarism. Isr J Psychiat and Rel Sci (1981)
18(4):283–297.

00220 ARNS, W.; WAHLE, H.
Über Die Dauerschäden Des Nervensystems Nach Einer
Fleckfieberenzephalitis. [*On Permanent Damages of the Nervous
System after a Typhus-Encephalitis*]. Fortschritte Der Neurol Psychiat
(1965) 33:113–144.

00230 ASKEVOLD, F.
Gibt Es Ein Generelles Kriegsschadensyndrom? [*Does a General War
Damage Syndrome Exist?*] In Cah d'inf Méd soc jurid (1983)
19:155–157.

00240 ASLANOV, A.
Die Rolle Der Störungen Der Tätigkeit Des Höheren Nervensystems
In Der Pathogenese Der Neuro-Psychischen Folgen Der Deportation
In Den Nazikonzentrationslagern (Störungen Festgestellt Bei
Deportierten Und Kriegsgefangenen). [*The Role of Disturbances of
Higher Nervous System Functions in the Pathogenesis of Neuro-Psychic
Sequels of Deportation in the Nazi Concentration Camps* (Disturbances
Determined in Deported persons and Prisoners of War)]. In
Ätio-Pathogenese Und Therapie Der Erschöpfung Und Vorzeitigen

Vergriesung. IV Internationaler Medizinischer Kongress. Bucharest: Verlag Der F.I.R., 1964, 584–591.

00250 AUERHAHN, N.C.; PRELINGER, E.
Repetition in the Concentration Camp Survivor and Her Child. Int Rev Psychoanal (1983) 10(1):31–46.

00251 AUERHAHN, N.C.; LAUB, D.
Annihilation and Restoration: Post-Traumatic Memory as Pathway and Obstacle to Recovery. Int Rev Psychoanal (1984) 11:327–344.

00260 AXELROD, S.; SCHNIPPER, O.L.; RAU, J.H.
Hospitalized Offspring of Holocaust Survivors. Problems and Dynamics. Bull Menninger Clinic (1980) 44(1):1–14.

00270 AYALON, O.; EITINGER, L.; LANSEN, J.; SUNIER, A.
The Holocaust and Its Perseverance, Stress, Coping and Disorder. Sinai-series 2, Van Gorcum (ed.). Assen, Holland, 1983.

00280 BAEYER, Von, W.R.; KISKER, K.P.
Abbiegung Der Persönlichkeitsentwicklung Eines Jugendlichen Durch Nationalsocialistische Verfolgungen. Paranoide Fehlhaltung. [*Deviations in the Development of the Personality of a Juvenile Caused by National-Socialistic Persecution. Paranoid Maladjustment*]. In March, H. (ed.), Verfolgung Und Angst. Stuttgart: Ernst Klett Verlag, 1960, 11–27.

00290 BAEYER, Von, W.R.
Erlebnisbedingte Verfolgungsschäden. [*Damage Caused by Experienced Persecution*]. Nervenarzt (1961) 32(12):534–538.

00300 BAEYER, Von, W.R.; HÄFNER, H; KISKER, K.P.
"Wissenschaftliche Erkenntnis" Oder "Menschliche Wertung" Der Erlebnisreaktiven Schäden Verfolgter. [*"Scientific Insight" or "Human Evaluation" of Damage Caused by Experienced Persecution*]. Nervenartz (1963) 34(3):120–123.

00310 BAEYER, Von, W.R.
Social and Political Aspects of Anxiety. Manuscript.

00320 BAEYER, Von, W.R.; HÄFNER, H.; KISKER, K P.
Zur Frage Des "Symptomfreien Intervalles" Bei Erlebnisreaktiven Störungen Verfolgter. [*On the Problem of the "Symptomless Interval" of Disturbances Caused by Persecution*]. In Paul, H., and H.J. Herberg (eds.), Psychische Spätschäden Nach Politischer Verfolgung. Basel: S. Karger, 1963, 125–153.

00330 BAEYER, Von, W.R.; HÄFNER, H.; KISKER, K.P.
Psychiatrie Der Verfolgten. [*The Psychiatry of the Persecuted*]. Berlin: Springer Verlag, 1964.

00340 BAEYER, Von, W.R.
Über Die Auswirkungen Der Verfolgung Und Konzentrationslagerhaft Vom Standpunkt Des Psychiaters. [*On the Effect of Persecution and Concentration Camp Internment From the Point of View of the*

Psychiatrist]. In Herberg, H. J. (ed.), Spätschäden Nach
Extrembelastungen. II Internationalen Medizinisch-Juristischen
Konferenz in Düsseldorf, 1969. Herford: Nicolaische
Verlagsbuchhandlung, 1971, 176–181.

00350   BAEYER, Von, W. R.
Über Die Entstehung Der Schizophrenie Ist Ein Wandel Der Früher
Herrschenden Lehrmeinung Eingetreten. Zur Frage, Wann Einer
Schizophrenie Als Verfolgungsleiden Anerkannt Werden Kann. [*A
Change of Opinion about the Development of Schizophrenia Has
Emerged, as in Contrast to the Formerly Prevailing Theory*].
Entscheidungen Der Bundesrepublik (1976) 2:49–50.

00360   BAEYER, Von, W. R.
[*On the Pathogenetic Significance of Extreme Psychosocial Stress in the
Development of Endogenous Psychoses*]. (Author's Trans). Nervenarzt
(1977) 48(9):471–477.

00370   BAEYER, Von W. R.; BINDER, W.
Endomorphe Psychosen Bei Verfolgten. [*Endomorphic Psychoses in
Persecuted Persons. Statistical-Clinical Studies of Compensation
Judgments*]. Monogr Gesamtgeb Psychiatr Berlin: Springer Verlag
(1982) 29:1–185.

00380   BALAZ, V.; BALAZOVA, E.
Die Klinisch Physiologischen Mechanismen Der Gegenwärtigen
Aktiven Folgen Des Krieges Für Die Gesundheit Der
Widerstandskämpfer Und Die Damit Verbundenen Therapeutischen
Probleme. [*The Effect of Clinical Physiological Mechanisms of
Contemporary Active War Sequelae, on the Health of Resistance Fighters
and the Therapeutic Problems Connected with Them*]. IV
Internationaler Medizinischer Kongress Der F.I.R., Prague, 1976.

00390   BARAB, G.
Tguvot Meuharot Etsel Meshuhrarei Mahanot Rikuz. [*Belated
Reactions in Former Concentration Camp Inmates.*] Harefuah (1956)
50:228–229.

00400   BARDIGE, B. S.
*Reflective Thinking and Prosocial Awareness: Adolescents Face the
Holocaust and Themselves.* Dissertation Abstracts International (1983)
44(5-B):1614.

00410   BARNHOORN, J. A. J.
Verhongering als mogelijke oorzaak van nerveuse, psychische en
psychosomatische stoornissen. [*Starvation as a Possible Cause of
Nervous, Psychic and Psychosomatic Disturbances*]. The Hague:
Buitengewone Pensioenraad, 1954.

00420   BAROCAS, H. A.
A Note on the Children of Concentration Camp Survivors. Psychother
(1971) 8:189–190.

00430 BAROCAS, H.A.; BAROCAS, C.B.
Manifestations of Concentration Camp Effects on the Second Generation. Am J Psychiat (1973) 130(7):820– 821.

00440 BAROCAS, H.A.
Children of Purgatory: Reflections on the Concentration Camp Survival Syndrome. Int J Soc Psychiat (1975) 21(2):87– 92.

00450 BAROCAS, H.A.; BAROCAS, C.B.
Wounds of the Fathers: The Next Generation of Holocaust Victims. Int Rev Psychoanal (1979) 6:331– 341.

00460 BAROCAS, H.A.; BAROCAS, C.B.
Separation-Individuation Conflicts in Children of Holocaust Survivors. J Contemp Psychother (1980) 11(1):6– 14. (Special Issue).

00470 BARON, L.
Surviving the Holocaust. J Psychol Judaism (1977) 1(2):25– 37.

00480 BARRAL, P.
Behandlung Des Konzentrationslagersyndroms Und Der Allgemeinen Mangelzustände Durch Die Fraktion "B" Des Serums, [*Treatment of the Concentration Camp Syndrome and General States of Deficiencies with Fraction "B" of the Serum*]. In Die Behandlung Der Asthenie Und Der Vorzeitigen Vergreisung Bei Ehemaligen Widerstanskämpfern Und KZ Häftlingen. III Internationale Medizinische Konferenz. Liège: Verlag Der F.I.R., 1961, 165– 185.

00490 BASTIAANS, J.
Psychosomatische gevolgen van onderdrukking en verzet. [*Psychosomatic Sequelae of Persecution and Resistance*]. Amsterdam: Noord-Hollandsche Uitgevers Maatschappij, 1957.

00500 BASTIAANS, J.
The Role of Aggression in the Genesis of Psychosomatic Disease. Psychosom Res (1969) 13:307– 314.

00510 BASTIAANS, J.
Over de specificiteit en de behandeling van het KZ-Syndroom. [*On the Specifics and the Treatment of the Concentration Camp Syndrome*]. Ned Mil Geneesk Tijdschr (1970) 23:364– 371.

00520 BASTIAANS, J.
General Comments on the Role of Aggression in Human Psychopathology. In Psychotherapy and Psychosomatics (eds. J. Ruesch, A.H. Schmale, Th. Spoerri) Basel: Karger, 1972. 20:300– 311.

00530 BASTIAANS, J.
Oorlogsleed in soorten. [*Types of Sorrow Caused by the War*]. In Life After a War: A Package of Information on the Working Through of Experiences from the War 1940– 1945. Utrecht, 1972. Manuscript.

00540 BASTIAANS, J.
Verlating en rouw. [*Desertion and Mourning*]. Intermediair 10 (1974) 20 (17– 5– 1974).

00550 BASTIAANS, J.
Het KZ syndroom en de menselijke vrijheid. [*The KZ Syndrome and Human Freedom*]. Ned Tijdschr Geneesk (1974) 118:1173–1178.

00560 BASTIAANS J.
The KZ Syndrome. A Thirty Year Study of the Effects on Victims of Nazi Concentration Camps. Rev Med Chir Soc Med Nat Iasi (1974) 78(3):573–578.

00570 BASTIAANS, J.
The Optimal Use of Anxiety in the Struggle for Adaptation. In Spielberger, C. D. and J. G. Sarason (eds.), Stress and Anxiety. New York: Wiley, 1977.

00580 BASTIAANS, J.
Control of Aggression and Psychotherapy. In Israel-Netherlands Symposium on the Impact of Persecution, Jerusalem, 1977. The Netherlands: Rijswijk, 1979, 25–37.

00590 BASTIAANS, J.
The Use of Hallucinogenic Drugs in Psychosomatic Therapy. Paper Read at the European Conference on Psychosomatic Research in Bodo, Norway, 1978. Manuscript.

00600 BASTIAANS, J.
De behandeling van oorlagsslachtoffers. [*The Treatment of War Victims*]. TGO Tijdschr Voor Geneesmiddelenonderzoek. J Drug Res (1979) 1:1–8.

00610 BASTIAANS, J.
Psychotherapy of War Victims Facilitated by the Use of Hallucinogenic Drugs. Read at the Vth World Congress of the International College of Psychosomatic Medicine, Jerusalem, 1979. Manuscript.

00620 BASTIAANS, J.
Vom Menschen Im KZ Und Vom KZ Im Menschen, Ein Beitrag zur Behandlung des KZ-Syndroms Und Dessen Spätfolgen. [*On People in the Concentration Camp and the Concentration Camp in People, A Lecture on the Management of Concentration Camp Syndromes and Their Consequences*] In Die Wiederkehr von Krieg und Verfolgung in Psychoanalysen, Hersg H. Henseler und A. Kuchenbuch, Ulm, Berlin, 1980.

00630 BASTIAANS, J.
De behandeling van oorlogsslachtoffers. [*The Treatment of War Victims*]. Arts en Wereld (1984) 17:(1)9–17.

00640 BAUMGARTEN-WESSEL, M. E.
Wet uitkeringen vervolgingsslachtoffers 1940–1945. [*The Compensation-Law for Persecuted People 1940–1945*]. Skriptie Rijksuniversiteit Leiden, Faculteit der Rechtsgeleerdheid (Faculty of Law Thesis). Leiden, 1977.

00650 BEARDWELL-WIELEZYNSKA, M.
[*The Concentration Camp in Bergen-Belsen Immediately after the Liberation*]. Przeglad Lekarski (1967) 23(1):105–112.

00660   BECKER, E.
The Pawnbroker: A Study in Basic Psychology. Angel in Armor. New
York: Free Press, Macmillan, 1969.

00670   BECKER M.
Extermination Camp Syndrome. New Eng J Med (1963) 268:1145.

00680   BEKKERING, P.G.
Kinderen als oorlogsslachtoffers. [*Children As War Victims*]. Ned
Tijdschr Geneesk (1981) 125(18):713–714.

00690   BELAISCH, J.
Die Hormontherapie Beim Deportierten Im Jahre 1961. [*The
Hormonal Therapy in Deportees in 1961*]. In Die Behandlung Der
Asthenie Und Der Vorzeitigen Vergreisung Bei Ehemaligen
Widerstanskämpfern Und KZ Häftlingen. III Internationale
Medizinische Konferenz. Liège: Verlag Der F.I.R., 1961, 101–106.

00700   BELLERT, J.
*The Polish Red Cross Camp Hospital After the Liberation of the Camp
in Auschwitz.* In Auschwitz, In Hell They Preserved Human Dignity,
Vol. 2, Part 2. Warsaw: International Auschwitz Committee, 1971.
123–143.

00710   BEN-BARUCH, M.
*Re-evaluation of the Right of Holocaust Survivors to Exist Through a
Social-Work Approach.* Israel-Netherlands Symposium on the Impact
of Persecution, 2. Dalfsen, Amsterdam, 14–18 April 1980. The
Netherlands: Rijswijk, 1981, 117–119.

00720   BENDINER, E.
Korczak: Pediatrician on the Road to Hell. Hosp Pract (1981)
16(7):125–128, 132–134, 138–139.

00730   BENNER, P.; ROSKIES, E.; LAZARUS, R.
Stress and Coping under Extreme Conditions. In Dimsdale, J.E. (ed.),
Survivors, Victims and Perpetrators. Washington: Hemisphere
Publishing, 1980, 219–258.

00740   BENSHEIM, H.
Die KZ-Neurose Rassich Verfolgter. Ein Beitrag Zur
Psychopathologie Der Neurosen. [*The Concentration Camp Neurosis of
Racially Persecuted Persons. A Contribution to the Psychopathology of
Neuroses*]. Nervenarzt (1960) 31:462–471.

00750   BEN-SIRA, Z.
*Loss, Stress and Readjustment: The Structure of Coping with
Bereavement and Disability.* Soc Sci Med (1983) 17(21):1619–1632.

00760   BEN-SIRA, Z.
Chronic Illness, Stress and Coping. Soc Sci Med (1984) 18(9):725–736.

00770   BEREZIN, M.A.
The Aging Survivor of the Holocaust. Introduction. J Geri Psychiat
(1981) 14(2):131–133.

00780   BEREZIN, M.A.; KAHANA, R.J.; PAYNE, E.C.
Psychotherapy of the Elderly. J Geri Psychiat (1983) 16(1):3–102.

00790   BENNER, P.; ROSKIES, E.; LAZARUS, R.S.
Stress and Coping under Extreme Conditions. In Dimsdale, J.E. (ed.),
Survivors, Victims and Perpetrators: Essays on the Nazi Holocaust.
New York: Hemisphere Publishing, 1980, 219–258.

00800   BERGER, D.E.
Children of Nazi Holocaust Surivivors: A Coming of Age. M.A. Thesis,
Goddard College, 1980. Manuscript at University of British
Columbia; Simon Wiesenthal Center Library of Los Angeles.

00810   BERGER, D.M.
The Survivor Syndrome: A Problem of Nosology and Treatment. Am J
Psychother (1977) 31(2):238–251.

00820   BERGHOFF, E.
Zum Begriff Der Sogenannten 'Lagerschäden' Und Deren
Auswirkungen. [*On the Concept of the So-Called "Camp Damages" and
Its Effects*]. In Ätio-Pathogenese Und Therapie Der Erschoepfung Und
Vorzeitigen Vergreisung. IV Internationaler Medizinischer Kongress.
Bucharest: Verlag Der F.I.R., 1964, 119–120.

00830   BERGMANN, M.S.; JUCOVY, M.E.
(Eds.) *Generations of The Holocaust.* New York: Basic Books, 1982.

00840   BERGMANN, M.S.
Recurrent Problems in the Treatment of Survivors and Their Children. In
Bergmann, M.S. and M.E. Jucovy (eds.), Generations of the
Holocaust. New York: Basic Books, 1982, 247–266.

00850   BERGMANN, M.S.; and JUCOVY, M.E.
Thoughts on Superego Pathology of Survivors and Their Children. In
Bergmann, M.S. and M.E. Jucovy (eds.), Generations of the
Holocaust. New York: Basic Books, 1983, 287–309.

00860   BERGMANN, M.S.
*Therapeutic Issues in the Treatment of Holocaust Survivors and Their
Children.* Am J Soc Psychiat (1983) III, 1:21–23.

00870   BERGMANN, M.S.; FURST, S.; GROSSMANN, F.; WANGH, M.
Psychoanalysis and the Holocaust: A Roundtable. In Luel, S.A., and
P. Marcus (eds.), Psychoanalytic Reflections on the Holocaust:
Selected Essays. New York: Ktav Publishing House, 1984.

00880   BERL, F.
The Adjustment of Displaced Persons. Jew Ass Soc Serv Q (1948) 24,
254.

00890   BERMAN, A.
*The Fate of Children in the Warsaw Ghetto in the Catastrophe of
European Jewry.* (Eds: Y. Gutman and L. Rotkirchen) Jerusalem: Yad
Vashem, 1976.

00900   BEROU, L.; DIMITRIU, A.; IACOBINI, P.
Über Die Morbidität Ehemaliger Politischer Häftlinge, Verschleppter

Personen und Antifaschistischer Kämpfer Der Widerstandsbewegung In Der Rumänischen Volksrepublik Und Über Therapeutische Massnahmen Sozialen Charakters In Unserem Lande. [*On the Morbidity of Formal Political Prisoners, Deported Persons and Anti-Fascist Fighters of the Resistance Movement in the Rumanian Republic, and about Therapeutic Measures of Social Character in our Country*]. In Ätio-Pathogenese Und Therapie Der Erschöpfung Und Vorzeitigen Vergreisung. IV Internationaler Medizinischer Kongress. Bucharest: Verlag Der F.I.R., 1964, 573–578.

00910   BETTELHEIM, B.
Individual and Mass Behavior in Extreme Situations. J Abnormal and Soc Psychol (1943) 38:417–452.

00920   BETTELHEIM, B.
Surviving and Other Essays. New York: Knopf, 1979.

00930   BETZENDAHL, W.
Über Die Frage Der Spätfolgen Von Fleckfieber Und Wolhynienfieber. [*On the Problem of Late Sequelae of Typhus and of Trench-Fever*]. Allg Zscbchr Psychiat (1949) 124:130–161.

00940   BIALONSKI, H.
Das Rehabilitationswesen Im In-Und Ausland. [*The Rehabilitation System in the Country and Abroad*]. In Schench, E. G. und W. Von Nathusius, Extreme Lebensverhältnisse Und Ihre Folgen. Germany: Verband Der Heimkehrer, 1959, Band 8, 70–96.

00950   BIALOWNA, I.
[*The Brzezinka Concentration Camp and Its Hospital for Women*]. Przeglad Lekarski (1979) 36(1):164–175.

00960   BIBERSTEIN, A.
[*A Contribution to the History of the Krakow-Plaszow Nazi Concentration Camp*]. Przeglad Lekarski (1977) 34(1):195–198.

00970   BIERMANN, G.; BIERMANN, R.
Kinder In Israel. Prax Kinderpsychol Kinder-Psychiat (1967) 16:3:97–112.

00980   BIERMANN, G.
Identitätsprobleme Jüdischer Kinder und Jugendlicher in Deutschland. [*Identity Problems of Jewish Children and Youth in Germany*]. Prax Kinderpsychol (1964) 6:213.

00990   BILIKIEWICZ, T.
Reflections on the Psychology of Genocide. In Auschwitz, Inhuman Medicine, Anthology, Vol. 1, Part 1, Warsaw: International Auschwitz Committee, 1970.

01000   BLAHA, F.
Kriegsfolgen An Menschlicher Gesundheit In Der Tschechoslowakischen Sozialistischen Republik Aus Den Jahren 1938–1945. [*War Results on Persons' Health in the Czechoslovakian Republic of the Years 1938–1945*]. In Die Behandlung Der Asthenie

und Der Vorzeitigen Vergreisung Bei Ehemaligen
Widerstandskämpfern Und KZ Häftlingen. III Internationale
Medizinische Konferenz. Liège: Verlag Der F.I.R., 1961, 239–240.

01010   BLAHA, F.
Arteriosklerose. [*Arteriosclerosis*]. In Die Behandlung Der Asthenie
Und Der Vorzeitigen Vergreisung Bei Ehemaligen
Widerstandskämpfern Und KZ Häftlingen. III Internationale
Medizinische Konferenz. Liège: Verlag Der F.I.R., 1961, 81–82.

01020   BLAHA, F.
Folgen Des Krieges Für Die Menschliche Gesundheit Nach 20 Jahren.
[*Effects of the War on Human Health 20 Years Later*]. In Ätio-
Pathogenese Und Therapie Der Erschöpfung Und Vorzeitigen
Vergreisung. IV Internationaler Medizinischer Kongress Der F.I.R.
Bucharest: Verlag Der F.I.R., 1964, 241–244.

01030   BLAHA, F.
Folgen Des Krieges Für Die Menschliche Gesundheit. [*Sequelae of the
War on Human Health*]. In Ätio-Pathogenese Und Therapie Der
Erschöpfung Und Vorzeitigen Vergreisung. IV Internationaler
Medizinischer Kongress. Bucharest: Verlag Der F.I.R., 1964, 121–241.

01040   BLAHA, F.
Arteriosklerose, Hypertension Und Herzinfarkt Bei
Kriegsbeschädigten. [*Arteriosclerosis, Hypertension and Myocardial
Infarction in War Injured*]. In Herberg, H.J. (ed.), Spätschäden Nach
Extremebelastungen. II Internationalen Medizinische-Juristischen
Konferenz in Düsseldorf, 1969. Herford: Nicolaische
Verlagsbuchhandlung, 1971, 109–114.

01050   BLAHA, F.
Ärztliche Und Soziale Beurteilung Und Wiedergutmachung Der
Spätfolgen Durch Den 2. Weltkrieg Auf Den Gesundheitszustand
Nach 20 Jahren. [*Medical and Social Evaluation and Restitution of
Sequelae of the 2nd World War, on the State of Health After 20 Years*].
In Ermüdung Und Vorzeitiges Altern. Folge Von
Extremebelastungen. V Internationaler Medizinischer Kongress Der
F.I.R., Paris, 1970. Leipzig: Johann Ambrosius, 1973, 302–308.

01060   BLAHA, F.
Folgen Des 2. Weltkrieges Auf Den Gesundheitszustand. [*Sequelae of
the 2nd World War on the State of Health*]. In Ermüdung Und
Vorzeitiges Altern. Folge Von Extremebelastungen. V Internationaler
Medizinischer Kongress Der F.I.R., Paris, 1970. Leipzig: Johann
Ambrosius, 1973, 289–292.

01070   BLAU, D.; KAHANA, J.
(Eds.). *The Aging Survivor of the Holocaust.* (Special Issue.) J Geri
Psychiat (1981) 14(2).

01080   BLOCH, H.A.
The Personality of Inmates of Concentration Camps. Am J Socio (1947)
52:335–341.

01085   BLOCH, M. B.
Het post-concentratie Kampsyndroom. [*The Concentration Camp Syndrome*] Ned. Milit. Geneesk. T. (1971) 24:165.

01090   BLOKHIN, V. N.
Die Rückkehr Der Invaliden Des Vaterländischen Krieges In Das Berufsleben Der USSR. [*The Return of the Invalids of the Patriotic War into Professional Life in the USSR*]. In Michel, M. (ed.), Gesundheitsschäden Durch Verfolgung Und Gefangenschaft Und Ihre Spätfolgen. Frankfurt Am Main: Röderberg Verlag, 1955, 228–235.

01100   BLOS, P.
Children of Social Catastrophe. Sequelae in Survivors and the Children of Survivors. Minutes of discussion group 7. Meeting of the Am Psychoanal Ass NY, 1968.

01110   BLUHM, O. H.
How Did They Survive? Mechanism of Defense in Nazi Concentration Camps. Am J Psychother (1948) 2:3–32.

01120   BLUMENTHAL, N. N.
Factors Contributing to Varying Levels of Adjustment among Children of Holocaust Survivors. (Ph.D. diss., Adelphi University, 1981). Page 1596 in Vol. 42/04-B of Dissertation Abstracts International. Order No: AAD81-20876.

01130   BODER, D. P.
The Impact of Catastrophe: Assessment and Evaluation. J Psychol (1954) 38:3–50.

01140   BODER, D. P.
I Did Not Interview The Dead. Champaign: University of Illinois Press, 1949.

01150   BOEHME, Von, H.; SCHARKOFF, T.; SCHARKOFF, H.
Spätschäden Nach Abnormalen Lebensbedingungen. [*Late Sequelae of Abnormal Life Conditions*]. Zeitschrift Für Alternsforschung (1969) 22:55–68.

01160   BOEKEN, N.
Psychosocial Care of Victims of Persecution in the Netherlands. In Israel-Netherlands Symposium on the Impact of Persecution, Jerusalem, 1977. The Netherlands: Rijswijk, 1979, 45–61.

01170   BOEKEN, N.
Material Aspects of Private and Governmental Services. Israel-Netherlands Symposium on the Impact of Persecution 2, Dalfsen, Amsterdam, 14–18 April 1980. The Netherlands: Rijswijk, 1981.

01180   BOGUSZ, J.
Experiments Conducted by Nazi Physicians with University Degrees. In Auschwitz, Inhuman Medicine, Anthology, Vol. 1, Part 1. Warsaw: International Auschwitz Committee, 1970, 36–42.

01190   BOGUSZ, J.
[*Concentration Camps. Foreword*]. Przeglad Lekarski (1974)·
31(1):3–12.

01200   BOGUSZ, J.
Polnische Errungenschaften In Der Erforschung Medizinischer
Probleme Der Nazi-Okkupationszeit. [*Polish Achievements in the
Research of Medical Problems of the Nazi Occupation*]. VI
Internationaler Medizinischer Kongress Der F.I.R., Prague, 1976.

01210   BOGUSZ, J.
[*17th Issue Dedicated to Medical Problems during the Nazi Occupation:
Foreword*]. Przeglad Lekarski (1977) 34(1):3–16.

01220   BOGUSZ, J.
[*History of German Concentration Camps during World War II.
Introduction*]. Przeglad Lekarski (1978) 35(1):3–15.

01230   BOGUSZ, J.
[*Remarks of a Physician about the Martyrdom of the Polish Jews*].
Przeglad Lekarski (1984) 41(1):54–62.

01240   BONDY, C.
Problems of Internment Camps. Am J Abnormal and Soc Psychol
(1943) 38:453–475.

01250   BONDY, C.
Versagungstoleranz Und Versagungssituation. [*Psychological
Situations and Threshold of "Breakdown"*]. In Paul, H., and
H.J. Herberg (eds.), Psychische Spätschäden Nach Politischer
Verfolgung. Basel: S. Karger, 1963, 7–19.

01260   BONNARD, A.
*Some Discrepancies between Perception and Affect as Illustrated by
Children in Wartime.* Psychoanal Study of the Child (1954) 9:242–251.

01270   BORK, Van J.J.
Lichamelijke klachten bij volwassenen in mogelijk verband met
psychotraumatische belevenissen in de vroege jeugd. [*Physical
Complaints in Adults and the Possible Connection with
Psychotraumatic Events in Early Childhood*]. Lecture, Dutch
Psychoanalytic Association, 19 March 1977.

01280   BORKOWSKI, W.
[*Reminiscences From the "Sick Ward": In Auschwitz*]. Przeglad
Lekarski (1984) 41(1):100–108.

01290   BOUCHER, M.
Chronische Asthenie Und Flecktyphusrezidive Bei Den Ehemaligen
Deportierten (Brill'sche Krankheit). [*Chronic Asthenia and Recurrent
Typhus in Deportees* (Brill's Disease)]. In Ätio-Pathogenese Und
Therapie Der Erschöpfung Und Vorzeitigen Vergreisung. IV
Internationaler Medizinischer Kongress Der F.I.R., 1964, 85–87.

01300   BRAUN, A.
Some Remarks on Persecution Pathology. Psychother Psychosom (1974)
24:106–108.

01310 BRAININ, E.; KAMINER, I.J.
Psychoanalyse und Nationalsozialismus. [*Psychoanalysis and National Socialism*]. Psyche (1982) 36(11):989–1012.

01320 BREZNITZ, T.
Recent Stress and Bereavement in Israel. In Israel-Netherlands Symposium on the Impact of Persecution. Jerusalem, 1977. The Netherlands: Rijswijk, 1979, 76–80.

01330 BRIEGER, G.H.
The Medical Profession. In H. Friedlander and S. Milton (eds.), The Holocaust: Ideology, Bureaucracy and Genocide. Millwood, N.Y.: Kraus International, 1980, 141–150.

01340 BRODY, S.
The Son of a Refugee. The Psychoanalytic Study of the Child. New Haven: Yale University Press, 1973, 28:169–191.

01350 BROESSE-STRAUSS, I.; STEFFEN, H.
Zur Psychopathologie Von Kindern NS-Verfolgter Eltern. Zwei Psychosomatische Fallstudien. [*About the Psychopathology of Children of National-Socialistic Persecuted Parents*]. Kinder Und Jugendpsychiat (1976) 4(1):55–70.

01360 BROST, U.
Zur Praxis Der Wiedergutmachung. [*On The Practice of Reparations*]. In Herberg, H.J. (ed.), Die Beurteilung Von Gesundheitsschäden Nach Gefangenschaft Und Verfolgung. Internationalen Medizinisch-Juristischen Symposiums in Köln, 1967. Herford: Nicolaische Verlagsbuchhandlung, 1967, 73–76.

01370 BROST, U.
Beziehungen Von Ernahrung Und Arbeit Zur Haufigkeit Des Diabetes; Aufgezeigt An Todesursachenstatistiken. [*The Relationship of Nutrition and Work to the Frequency of Diabetes; Demonstrated on Statistics of Death*]. In Ermüdung und Vorzeitiges Altern: Folge von Extrembelastungen. V Internationaler Medizinischer Kongress Der F.I.R., Paris, 1970. Leipzig: Johann Ambrosius, 1973, 33–37.

01380 BROZEK, K.
[*Dr. Jan Buzek*]. Przeglad Lekarski (1980) 37(1):187–189.

01390 BRÜLL, F.
The Trauma: A Theoretical Consideration. Isr Ann Psychiat (1969–70):96–108.

01400 BRUGGEMAN, J.A.
Tweede generatie oorlogsslachtoffers. [*The Second Generation War Victims*]. In Frijling-Schreuder, B. (ed.), Psychoanalytici aan het Woord. Deventer, 248–257, 1980.

01410 BUSCHBOM, H.
Die Volkerrechtlichen Und Staatsrechtlichen Masznahmen Zur Beseitigung Des Im Namen Des Deutschen Reiches Verubten Nationalsozialistischen Unrechts. [*The Measures According to International Law and Constitutional Law in Order to Eliminate The*

National Socialist Injustice Caused in the Name of the German Reich]. In Die Wiedergutmachung Nationalsozialistischen Unrechts Durch Die Bundesrepublik Deutschland. Distributed by the Bundesminister of Finance in Collaboration with Walter Schwartz, Band 2. Munich, 1981, 1–73.

01420   BRYM, H.; LØNNUM, A.; OYEN, O.
Über Die Neuen Kriegspensionierungsgesetze In Norwegen. [*On the New War Pension In Norway*]. In Herberg, H.J. (ed.), Spätschäden Nach Extremebelastungen. II Internationalen Medizinisch-Juristischen Konferenz in Düsseldorf, 1969. Herford: Nicolaische Verlagsbuchhandlung, 1971, 311–316.

01430   BRZEZICKI, E.; GAWALEWICZ, A.; HOLUJ, T.; KEPINSKI, A.; KLODZINSKI, S.; WOLTER, W.
[*Prisoners with a Function in Nazi Concentration Camps (A Discussion)*]. Przeglad Lekarski (1968) 24(1):253–261.

01440   BULKA, R.P.
Editor's Perspective. J Psychol Judaism (1981) 6(1):5–6.

01450   BUNDY, J.
Wplyw Przebywania W Obozie Koncentracyjnym Na Uzebienie Bylych Wiezniow. [*The Influence of the Stay in a Concentration Camp on the Dental Status of Ex-Prisoners*]. Przeglad Lekarski (1968) 25:65–70.

01460   BUNDY, J.
Dentition of Former Prisoners. In Auschwitz, Anthology, Vol. 3, Part 2. Warsaw: International Auschwitz Committee, 1972, 42–80.

01470   BURES, R.
Fürsorge Für Die Invaliden Der Faschistischen Verfolgung In Der Tschechoslowaskischen Republik. [*Care for the Infirm Survivors of Fascist Persecution in the Republic of Czechoslovakia*]. In Michel, M. (ed.), Gesundheitsschäden Durch Verfolgung Und Gefangenschaft Und Ihre Spätfolgen. Frankfurt Am Main: Röderberg Verlag, 1955, 240–245.

01480   BURGMANN, W.
Fehlurteile Durch Überwertung Des Alkohols Als Ursache Von Leberkrankheiten, Speziell Cerebralen Erscheinungen Bei Zirrhose. [*False Judgement due to Overestimation of Alcohol as Cause of Liver Diseases, Particularly With Respect to Brain Symptoms in Cases of Cirrhosis*]. In Herberg, H.J. (ed.), Spätschäden Nach Extremebelastungen. II Internationalen Medizinisch-Juristischen Konferenz in Düsseldorf, 1969. Herford: Nicolaische Verlagsbuchhandlung, 1971, 229–236.

01490   BUSCH, M.D.
The Legacy of Affliction. An Enquiry into the Intergenerational Transmission of Social Pathology and Its Treatment amongst Nazi Concentration Camp Survivors and Their Children. MSW thesis, University of British Columbia, 1978.

01500 BYCHOWSKI, G.
       Permanent Character Changes as an Aftereffect of Persecution. In
       Krystal, H. (ed.), Massive Psychic Trauma. New York: International
       Universities Press, 1968, 75– 86.

01510 CANIVET, F.
       Myokardschäden. [*Damages of the Myocardium*]. In Michel, M. (ed.),
       Gesundheitsschäden Durch Verfolgung Und Gefangenschaft Und Ihre
       Spätfolgen. Frankfurt Am Main: Röderberg Verlag, 1955, 191.

01520 CAPINSKA, K.; CAPINSKI, T. Z.
       Wyniki Ambulatoryjnego Badania Dermatologicznego 150 Bylych
       Wiezniow Oswiecimia. [*The Results of a Dermatological Investigation
       of 150 Former Prisoners of Auschwitz*]. Przeglad Lekarski (1969)
       26:31– 35.

01530 CAPINSKA, K; CAPINSKI, T. Z.
       Ergebnisse Der Ambulaenten Dermatologischen Untersuchung Von
       150 Ehmaligen Auschwitz-Häftlingen 23 Jahre Nach Der Befreiung.
       [*Results of Dermatological Ambulatory Examinations of 150 Former
       Auschwitz Inmates 23 Years after Liberation*]. In Ermüdung Und
       Vorzeitiges Altern. Folge Von Extremebelastungen. V Internationaler
       Medizinischer Kongress Der F.I.R., Paris, 1970. Leipzig: Johann
       Ambrosius, 1973, 158– 163.

01540 CAPINSKA, K.; CAPINSKI, T. Z.; PIECHOCKI, M.
       Dalsze Wyniki Ogolnopolskich Dermatlogicznych Badan Bylych
       Wiezniow. [*Further Results of an "All Poland" Dermatological
       Investigation of Ex-Prisoners*]. Przeglad Lekarski (1978) 35:27– 29.

01550 CARMELLY, F.
       *Guilt Feelings in Concentration Camp Survivors: Comments of a
       "Survivor."* J Jewish Comm Serv (1975) 52(2):139– 144.

01560 CARMON, A.
       *Summary of the Introduction on the Role of the School in Relation to
       Education in Families, Schools and Other Settings.* Israel-Netherlands
       Symposium on the Impact of Persecution 2. Dalfsen, Amsterdam.
       14– 18 April 1980. The Netherlands: Rijswijk, 1981. 105, 106– 108.

01570 CATH, S. H.
       *The Aging Survivor of the Holocaust. Discussion: The Effects of the
       Holocaust on Life-Cycle Experiences: The Creation and Recreation of
       Families.* J Geri Psychiat (1981) 14(2):155– 163.

01580 CESA-BIANCHI, M.; DEVOTO, A.; MARTINI, M.
       *Psychopathological Consequences of Internment in Nazi Concentration
       Camps.* VI internationaler Medizinischer Kongress Der F.I.R., Prague,
       1976.

01590 CHODOFF, P.
       *Effects of Extreme Coercive and Oppressive Forces: Brainwashing and
       Concentration Camps.* In Arieti, S. (ed.), American Handbook of
       Psychiatry. New York: Basic Books, 1959, 384– 405.

01600   CHODOFF, P.
Late Effects of the Concentration Camp Syndrome. Arch Gen Psychiat
(1963) 8:323– 333.

01610   CHODOFF,P.
Nazi Concentration Camp Survivors—Still Inmates. Roche Report:
Frontiers of Clinical Psychiatry (1966) 3(4).

01620   CHODOFF, P.
*The Nazi Concentration Camp and the American Poverty Ghetto—A
Comparison.* J Contemp Psychother (1968) 1:1– 8.

01630   CHODOFF, P.
Depression and Guilt among Concentration Camp Survivors.
Existential Psychiat (1970) 7:19– 26.

01640   CHODOFF, P.
The German Concentration Camp as a Psychological Stress. Arch Gen
Psychiat (1970) 22(1):78– 87.

01650   CHODOFF, P.
Psychological Response to Concentration Camp Survival. In H. Abram
(ed.), Psychological Aspects of Stress. Springfield, Ill: Thomas, 1970.

01660   CHODOFF, P.
Psychiatric Aspects of the Nazi Persecution. In Arieti, S. (ed.), Am H
Psychiat. New York: Basic Books (1975) 41:932– 946.

01670   CHODOFF, P.
Psychotherapy of the Survivor. In Dimsdale, J. E. (ed.), Survivors,
Victims and Perpetrators. Washington: Hemisphere Publishing, 1980,
205– 216.

01680   CHODOFF, P.
Survivors of the Nazi Holocaust.   Children Today (1981) 10:2– 6.

01690   CHYLINSKA, M.
[*Defence Mechanisms*]. Przeglad Lekarski (1984) 41(1):121– 126.

01700   CITROME, P.
Conclusions d'une Enquête sur le Suicide dans les Camps de
Concentration. [*Conclusions of a Study on Suicide in Concentration
Camps*]. Cah Int Sociol (1952) 12:147– 149.

01710   CIUCA, A.
La Pathologie Sequellaire (après L'age de 30 Ans) des Résistants.
[*The Pathological Sequelae (after 30 Years of Age) in Resistance
Fighters*]. VI Congrès Médical International de la F.I.R., Prague, 1976.

01720   COHEN, E.A.
Het duitse concentratie-kamp. Een medische en psychologische
studie. [*The German Concentration Camp. A Medical and Psychological
Study*]. Amsterdam: H.J. Paris, 1952.

01730   COHEN, E.A.
Human Behavior in the Concentration Camp. New York: Universal
Library, 1953.

01740   COHEN, E. A.
Reakcja Poczatkowa Na Osadzenie W Obozie Koncentracyjnym. [*The Primary Reaction to Imprisonment in Concentration Camps.*]. Przeglad Lekarski (1965) 21:28–31.

01750   COHEN, E. A.
KZ-Nachbar Der Inneren Grenze. Das Post-Konzentration-slager-Syndrom. [*The Post Concentration Camp Syndrome*]. in Areopag: Politisch Literarisches Forum. (Deutschland Und Seine Nachbarn) (1969) 213–218. Also in Polish: Przeglad Lekarski (1972) 29:1–7.

01760   COHEN, E. A.
Het Post-Concentratiekampsyndroom. [*The Post Concentration-Camp Syndrome*]. Ned Tijdschr Geneesk (1969) 113(46):2049–2054.

01770   COHEN, E. A.
Uwagi O Tzw KZ-Syndromie. [*On the So-called KZ Syndrome*]. Przeglad Lekarski (1972) 29:21–27.

01780   COHEN, E. A.
W Transporcie Wieznow-Zydow Z Holandii. [*On a Transport of Jewish Prisoners from Holland*]. Przeglad Lekarski (1972) 29:120–132. Also in German: Durch Den Schornstein.

01790   COHEN, E. A.
Het Post-Concentratiekampsyndroom: Een "Disaster" Syndroom. [*The Post-Concentration Camp Syndrome*]. Ned Tijdschr Geneesk (1972) 116(38):1680–1685.

01800   COHEN E. A.
The Abyss. A Confession. New York: Norton, 1973.

01810   COHEN, E. A.
Onvoltooid verleden tijd. [*The Imperfect Past*]. De hulpverlening aan oorlogsvervolgden, skriptie Sociale Academie, Amsterdam, 1973.

01820   COHEN, E. A.
The Post Concentration Camp Syndrome: A Disaster Syndrome. VI Internationaler Medizinischer Kongress Der F.I.R., Prague, 1976, 1–10.

01830   COHEN, E. A.
De negentien treinen naar sobibor. [*The Nineteen Trains to Sobibor*]. Brussels: Elsevier, 1979.

01835   COHEN, J.
The Impact of Death and Dying on Concentration Camp Survivors. Advances in Thanatology (1977) 4(1):27–36.

01840   COKE, L. R.
Late Effects of Starvation. Med Serv J Can (1961) 17:313–324.

01850   COLLIS, W. R. F.
Belsen Camp: A Preliminary Report. Brit Med J (1945):814–816.

01860   COOPER, R. H.
        Concentration Camp Survivors: A Challenge for Geriatric Nursing. Nurs
        Clinic N Am (1979) 14(4):621–628.

01870   COOPMANS, M. J. A. M.
        Tweede generatie vervolgingsslachtoffers 1940–1945. Een casus,
        verslag van de eerste wetenschapdag, gehouden op 18 November
        1983 in de DR. H. v.d. Hoevenkliniek te Utrecht, [*Second Generations
        Victims of Persecution 1940–45*], A Case, Proceedings of the First
        Science Day, held on 18 November 1983. In Voordrachtenreeks
        Nederlandse Vereniging voor Psychiatrie, no. 4, Amsterdam, 56–95.

01880   COPELMAN, L. S.
        Studien Und Forschungen Über Die Pathogenese Und Die
        Behandlung Des Psycho-Somatischen Syndroms Der Deportierten.
        [*Studies and Research of the Pathogenesis and Treatment of the
        Psychosomatic Syndromes of Deportees*]. In Die Behandlung Der
        Asthenie Und Der Vorzeutigen Vergreisung Bei Ehemaligen
        Widerstanskämpfern Und KZ Häftlingen. III Internationale
        Medizinische Konferenz. Liège: Verlag Der F.I.R., 1961, 107–118.

01890   COPELMAN, L. S.
        Schizophrenie Im Rahmen Der Sozialpsychiatrie. [*Schizophrenia
        within the Framework of Social Psychiatry*]. In Ermüdung Und
        Vorzeitiges Altern. Folge Von Extremebelastungen. V Internationaler
        Medizinischer Kongress Der F.I.R., Paris, 1970. Leipzig: Johann
        Ambrosius, 1973, 139–148.

01900   COPELMAN, L. S.
        Spät Auftretende Neuroendokrinologische Folgen Der
        Konzentrationslager Im Lichte Von Stoffwechselstoerungen. [*Delayed
        Appearance of Neuroendocrinological Sequelae of Concentration Camps
        as Reflected in Metabolic Disturbances*]. In Ermüdung Und Vorzeitiges
        Altern. Folge Von Extremebelastungen. V Internationaler
        Medizinischer Kongress Der F.I.R., Paris, 1970. Leipzig: Johann
        Ambrosius, 1973, 139–148.

01910   COPELMAN, L. S.
        La Délinquance Juvenile chez l'Enfant Concentrationnaire. [*Juvenile
        Delinquency of the Concentration Camp Child*]. In VI Internationaler
        Medizinischer Kongress Der F.I.R., Prague, 1976.

01920   COPELMAN, L. S.
        L'Etat Actuel de Nos Connaissances sur l'Etiologie des Sequelles de
        Guerre. [*The Contemporary State of Our Knowledge About the Etiology
        of War Sequelae*]. In VI Congrès Médical International de la F.I.R.,
        Prague, 1976.

01930   CORCORAN, J. F. T.
        *The Concentration Camp Syndrome and USAF Vietnam Prisoners of
        War.* Psychiat Ann (1982) 12:991–994.

01940   CORDELL, M.
        Coping Behavior of Nazi Concentration Camp Survivors. Ph.D. diss.,

Pacific Graduate School of Psychology, 1980. Page 3883 in Vol. 41/10-B of Dissertation Abstracts International. Order No: AAD81–04638.

01950 CORMIER, B. M.
On the History of Men and Genocide. Presented at the Fifth International Criminological Congress, Montreal, 1965, 1–16.

01955 CRAWFORD, F.
Accounting for Genocide—Victims and Survivors of the Holocaust. Soc Sci Q (1980) 49:179.

01960 CRAWFORD, J. N.
Note From Canada. In *Later Effects of Imprisonment and Deportation.* International Conference Organized by the World Veterans Federation. The Hague: World Veterans Federation, 1961, 146–147.

01970 CREMERIUS, J.
Eine Kindertragödie. Psychose Oder Neurose. [*A Children's Tragedy. Psychosis or Neurosis.*]. In March, H. (ed.), Verfolgung Und Angst. Stuttgart: Ernst Klett Verlag, 1960, 28–33.

01980 CREMERIUS, J.
Schiksal Und Neurose. Multiple Leib-Seelische Störungen Nach KZ-Haft. [*Fate and Neurosis. Multiple Physical-Mental Disturbances after Concentration Camp Imprisonment*]. In March, H. (ed.), Verfolgung Und Angst. Stuttgart: Ernst Klett Verlag, 1960.

01990 DABROWSKI, S.; SCHRAMMOWA, H.; ZAKOWSKA-DABROWSKA, T.
Trwale Zmiany Pschiczne Powstale W. Wyniku Pobytu W Obozach Koncentrcyjnych I Eksperymentow Pseudolekarskich. [*Persistent Psychological Changes Caused by Incarceration in a Concentration Camp and by Pseudomedical Experiments*]. In Piaty Zeszyt Poswiecony Zgadnieniom Lekarskim Okresu Hitlerowskiej Okupdcji. Przeglad Lekarski, (1965) 21(1):31–34.

02000 DADRIAN, V. N.
Factors of Anger and Aggression in Genocide. J Hum Rel (1971) 19(3):396–417.

02010 DAHMER, H.
Holocaust Und Die Amnesie. [*Holocaust and Amnesia*]. Psyche (1979) 33(11):1039–1049.

02020 DANE, J.
Keerzijde van de bevrijding, opstellen over de maatschappelijke, psycho-sociale en medische aspekten van de problematiek van oorlogsgetroffenen. [*The Reverse Side of the Liberation, Essays on the Social, Psychosocial and Medical Aspects of the Problems of War Victims*]. Deventer: Van Loghum Slaterus, 1984.

02030 DANGEL, J.
[*The Auschwitz and Dachau Concentration Camp Medical Centres*]. Przeglad Lekarski (1974) 31(1):209–213.

02040   DANIELI, Y.
Countertransference in the Treatment and Study of Nazi Holocaust
Survivors and Their Children. Second International Conference on
Psychological Stress and Adjustment in Time of War and Peace,
June, 1978, Jerusalem. In Victimology (1980) 5(2–4):355–367.

02050   DANIELI, Y.
Mit'am Hahitarvut Bedarcey Hahistaglut Hashonot Shel Mishpachot
Nitzoley Hashoa. [Fitting the Intervention to Different Modes of
Adaptation in Families of Survivors]. Masua (1981) 9:169–178.

02060   DANIELI, Y.
Differing Adaptational Styles in Families of Survivors of the Nazi
Holocaust. Some Implications for Treatment. Children Today (1981)
10(6–10):34–35.

02070   DANIELI, Y.
The Group Project for Holocaust Survivors and Their Children. Children
Today (1981) 10:11–13.

02080   DANIELI, Y.
Jewish Identity of Children of Survivors of the Nazi Holocaust.
Manuscript.

02090   DANIELI, Y.
The Aging Survivor of the Holocaust. Discussion: On the Achievement
of Integration in Aging Survivors of the Nazi Holocaust. J Geria
Psychiat (1981) 14(2):191–210.

02100   DANIELI, Y.
Therapists' Difficulties in Treating Survivors of the Nazi Holocaust and
Their Children. Ph.D. diss., New York University, 1981. Page 4927 in
Vol. 42/12-B of Dissertation Abstracts International. Order No:
AAD82–10968.

02110   DANIELI, Y.
On the Achievement of Integration in Aging Survivors of the Nazi
Holocaust. J Geri Psychiat (1981) 14(2):191–210.

02120   DANIELI, Y.
Families of Survivors of the Nazi Holocaust. Some Short and Long
Term Effects. In Milgram, N. (ed.), Stress and Anxiety. Washington:
Hemisphere Publishing, 1982, 405–421.

02130   DANIELI, Y.
Psychotherapists' Participation in the Conspiracy of Silence about the
Holocaust. Psychoanal Psychol (1983) 1:23–42.

02150   DANIELI, Y.
The Treatment and Prevention of Long Term Effects and
Intergenerational Transmission of Victimization: A Lesson from
Holocaust Survivors and Their Children. In Figley, C. R. (ed.), Trauma
and Its Wake. New York: Brunner Mazel, 1985.

02160   DANTO, B. L.
The Role of "Missed Adolescence" in the Etiology of the Concentration

Camp Survivor Syndrome. In Krystal, H. (ed.), Massive Psychic Trauma. New York: International Universities Press, 1968, 248–259.

02170 DAVID, H. P.
(Ed.). *Migration, Mental Health and Community Services.* Proceedings of a Conference Held in Geneva, 1966. Geneva: American Joint Distribution Committee, 1966.

02180 DAVID, J.
Pathology of the Captivity of the Prisoners of World War II. Works at the Int Med Conf, Brussels, 1962. Paris: Ed Int Confeder Ex-Prisoners of War, 1963.

02190 DAVIDSON, S.
A Clinical Classification of Psychiatric Disturbances of Holocaust Survivors and Their Treatment. Isr Ann Psychiat Rel Disc (1967) 5:96–98.

02200 DAVIDSON, S.
Tipul Benitsolei Shoah. [*A Classification of the Psychiatric Disturbances of Holocaust Survivors and Their Treatment*]. Manuscript, Dept. of Medicine, Kupath-Holim and Haifa University, 1974? An Expansion and Translation into Hebrew of the English Paper. Isr Ann Psychiat Rel Disc (1967) 5:96–98.

02210 DAVIDSON S.
Issues Concerning the Transmission of Psychopathology in Children of Concentration Camp Survivors. Presented to the San Francisco Psychoanalytic Institute, 23 February 1977. Manuscript.

02220 DAVIDSON, S.
Long-Term Psychosocial Sequelae in Holocaust Survivors and Their Families. In Israel-Netherlands Symposium on the Impact of Persecution, Jerusalem, 1977. The Netherlands: Rijswijk, 1979, 62–67.

02230 DAVIDSON, S.
Massive Psychic Traumatization and Social Support. J Psychosom Res (1979) 23:395–402.

02240 DAVIDSON, S.
The Clinical Effects of Massive Psychic Trauma in Families of Holocaust Survivors. J Mar and Fam Ther (1980) 6(1):11–21.

02250 DAVIDSON, S.
Transgenerational Transmission in the Families of Holocaust Survivors. Int J Fam Psychiat (1980) 1:95–112.

02260 DAVIDSON, S.
The Survivor Syndrome Today: An Overview. Group Analysis, Special Issue: The Survivor Syndrome Workshop (November 1980) 24–32.

02270 DAVIDSON, S.
On Relating to Traumatized-Persecuted People. Israel-Netherlands Symposium on the Impact of Persecution. 2, Dalfsen, Amsterdam, 14–18 April 1980. The Netherlands: Rijswijk, 1981, 55–62.

02280 DAVIDSON, S.
Le Syndrom de Survivants: Revue Generale. [*The Survivor's Syndrome: A General View*]. L'Evolution Psychiatr (1981) 46:321–331.

02290 DAVIDSON, S.
Nitzoley Hashoa Umishpachoteihem: Nisajon Klini Psychotherapeuti. [*Clinical and Psychotherapeutic Experience with Survivors and Their Families*]. Fam Physician (1981) 10(2):319–331.

02300 DAVIDSON, S.
Psychosocial Issues in the Lives of Survivors. J Aid Soc (1981) 29–33.

02310 DAVIDSON, S.
Psychosocial Aspects of Holocaust Trauma in the Life Cycle of Survivors-Refugees and Their Families. In Baker, R. (ed.), The Psychosocial Problems of Refugees. London, 1983. 21–31.

02320 DEBICKA-MALKOWSKA, D.; FOERSTERLING, E.; KINAL, K.; LEWANDOWSKA, M.
Wyniki Bydgoskick Badan Bylych Wiezniow Hitlerowskich Obozow Koncentracyjnych. [*The Results of the Investigations Performed in the County of Bydgoszcz of Former Prisoners in Hitlerian Concentration Camps*]. Przeglad Lekarski (1972) 29:23–34.

02330 DELIUS, L.
Pathogenese Und Prognose Vegetativer Regulationsstörungen. [*Pathogenesis and Prognosis of Disturbances in the Vegetative Regulation*]. In Extreme Lebensverhältnisse Und Ihre Folgen. Bericht Über Den 4 Ärtzekongress Für Pathologie. Therapie Und Begutachtung Der Heimkehrerkrankheiten In Düsseldorf, 1959. N.P.: Verband Der Heimkehrer, 1959, Band 8, 54–57.

02340 DENES, S.
Premature Aging and Invalidity. VI Internationaler Medizinischer Kongress Der F.I.R. Prague, 1976.

02350 DERSHOWITZ, N.H.
The Long-Range Effects of Concentration Camp Internment on Certain Variables of Personality, Cognitive and Perceptual Functioning on Nazi Victims, Their Children. Department of Psychology. Bar Ilan University. Ramat-Gan, 1972. Manuscript.

02360 DESMONTS, T.
Die Hautpigmentierung Bei Den KZ Insassen Während Und Nach Der Deportation. [*Pigmentation of the Skin in Concentration Camps Inmates during and after Deportation*]. In Michel, M. (ed.), Gesundheitsschäden Durch Verfolgung Und Gefangenschaft Und Ihre Spätfolgen. Frankfurt Am Main: Röderberg Verlag, 1955.

02370 DESMONTS, T.
Puls, Blutdruck Und Hungeroedem Bei 196 Politischen Deportierten. [*Pulse, Bloodpressure and Oedema Due to Famine in 196 Political Deportees*]. In Michel, M. (ed.), Gesundheitsschäden Durch Verfolgung Und Gefangenschaft Und Ihre Spätfolgen. Frankfurt Am Main: Röderberg Verlag, 1955.

02380 DESOILLE, H.
Berufliche Umschulung Der Kranken Ehemaligen Deportierten In
Frankreich. [*Vocational Reschooling of Ill People Formerly Deported in
France*]. In Michel, M. (ed.), Gesundheitsschäden Durch Verfolgung
Und Gefangenschaft Und Ihre Spätfolgen. Frankfurt Am Main:
Röderberg Verlag, 1955. Also In Fichez, L. (ed.), Andere Spätfolgen.
Austria: Verlag Der F.I.R., 1959, Band 2, 219–227.

02390 DESOILLE, H.
Hygiene Und Diät Für Ehemalige Deportierte. [*Hygiene and Diet For
Former Deportees*]. In Die Behandlung Der Asthenie Und Der
Vorzeitigen Vergreisung Bei Ehemaligen Widerstanskämpfern Und
KZ Häftlingen. III Internationale Medizinisch Konferenz. Liège:
Verlag Der F.I.R., 1961.

02400 DES-PRES, T.
The Survivor: On the Ethos of Survival in Extremity. Encounter (1971)
37:3–19.

02410 DES-PRES, T.
Survivors and the Will to Bear Witness. Soc Res (1973) 40:668–690.

02420 DES-PRES, T.
The Survivor: An Anatomy of Life in the Death Camps. New York:
Oxford University Press, 1976.

02430 DES-PRES, T.
Victims and Survivors. Dissent (1976) 23(1):49–56.

02440 DES-PRES, T.
The Lesson of Treblinka. Quest (1979) 3:15–18.

02450 DES-PRES, T.
The Bettelheim Problem. Soc Res (1979) 46(4):619–647.

02460 DESSAUR-FEIGENBAUM, R.
Brieven aan vaders en moeders, over de kinderen van
oorlogsslachtoffers: de tweede generatie. [*Letters to Fathers and
Mothers, on The Children of War Victims: The Second Generation*]. The
Hague, 1975.

02470 DESSAUR-FEIGENBAUM, R.
De tweede generatie. [*The Second Generation, Thesis*]. The Hague,
1984.

02480 DEVEEN, W.
Aetio-Pathogenese Und Therapie Der Erschöpfung Und Vorzeitigen
Vergreisung. [*Ethio-Pathogenesis and Therapy of Exhaustion and
Premature Aging*]. In Aetio-Pathogenese Und Therapie Der
Erschöpfung Und Vorzeitigen Vergreisung. IV Internationaler
Medizinischer Kongress Der F.I.R. Bucharest: Verlag Der F.I.R., 1964,
597–581.

02490 DEVEEN, W.
Die Rheumatischen Erkrankungen Bei Den Ehemaligen Deportierten.
[*Rheumatic Illness in Former Deportees*]. In Michel, M. (ed.),

Gesundheitsschäden Durch Verfolgung Und Gefangenschaft Und Ihre
Spätfolgen. Frankfurt Am Main: Röderberg Verlag, 1955, 198–208.
Also in Fichez, L. (ed.), Andere Spätfolgen. Austria: Verlag Der F.I.R.,
1959, Band 2, 154–158.

02500   DEVEEN, W.
Rheumatism and Deportation. In Later Effects of Imprisonment and
Deportation. International Conference Organized by the World
Veterans Federation. The Hague: World Veterans Federation, 1961,
79–82.

02510   DEVOTO, A.; BUFFULINI, A.; MARTINI, M.
Ergebnisse Einer Psychologischen Analyse, Durchgefurht An Einer
Gruppe Ehemaliger Italienischer KZ-Häftlinge. [Results of a
Psychological Analysis Held on a Group of Former Italian
Concentration Camp Inmates]. In Cah d'inf méd, soc jurid (1983)
19:67–69.

02520   DIAMANT, J.
Some comments on the Psychology of Life in the Ghetto Terezin. In
Terezin. Prague, 1965, 125–139.

02530   DICKHAUT, H. H.
Zur Frage Der Dauerschäden Nach Fleckfieberenzephalitis. [The
Problem of Permanent Damage after Typhus Encephalitis]. Fortsch
Neurol Psychiatr Hamburg (1959) 27:20–32.

02540   DICKHAUT, H. H.
Dauerschäden Nach Fleckfieber-Encephalits. [Permanent Disturbances
after Typhus Encephalitis]. In Herberg, H. J. (ed.), Spätschäden Nach
Extremebelastungen. II Internationalen Medizinisch-Juristischen
Konferenz in Düsseldorf, 1969. Herford: Nicolaische
Verlagsbuchhandlung, 1971, 200–202.

02550   DICKS, H. V.
Licensed Mass Murder: A Socio-psychological Study of Some SS Killers.
New York: Basic Books, 1972.

02560   DIETZE, A.
Begutachtung Und Beurteilung Von Leberschäden Nach Extremen
Lebensverhältnissen. [Examination and Evaluation of Liver Damage
after Extreme Life Situations]. In Herberg, H. J. (ed.), Die Beurteilung
Von Gesundheitsschäden Nach Gefangenschaft Und Verfolgung.
Internationalen Medizinisch-Juristischen Symposiums in Köln, 1967.
Herford: Nicolaische Verlagsbuchhandlung, 1967, 114–120.

02570   DIETZE, A.
Katamnestische Untersuchungen Bei Leber Krankheiten Ehemaliger
Gefangener. [Catamnestic Examinations in Former Prisoners with Liver
Diseases]. IV Internationaler Medizinischer Kongress Der F.I.R.,
Prague, 1976.

02580   DIGGELEN, Van, W.
Vervolgingsslachtoffers en de hulpverlening, vergelijk van
hulpverlening 'ter verbetering van de sociale omgeving' van joodse

vervolgingsslachtoffers in Polen en Nederland. [*Victims of Persecution and Assistance, Comparison of Assistance to Improve the Social Surroundings of Jewish Persecution Victims in Poland and Holland*]. Amsterdam, 1976.

02590 DIMSDALE, J. E.
The Coping Behavior of Nazi Concentration Camp Survivors. Am J Psychiat (1974) 131:792–797.

02600 DIMSDALE, J. E.
Coping: Every Man's War. Am J Psychother (1978) 32:402–413.

02610 DIMSDALE, J. E.
The Coping Behavior of Nazi Concentration Camp Survivors. In Dimsdale, J. E. (ed.), Survivors, Victims and Perpetrators. Washington: Hemisphere Publishing, 1980.

02620 DIMSDALE, J. E.
Survivors, Victims and Perpetrators. Washington: Hemisphere Publishing, 1980. With chapters by: Benner, Chodoff, Dimsdale, Hamburg, Eitinger, Lifton, Luchterhand, Russell.

02630 DOBRE, M.; CIUCA, A.; JORDANA, B.
Les Aspects Psychologiques du Viellissement chez un Groupe d'Anciens Combattants Antifascistes. [*The Psychological Aspects of Aging in a Group of Former Antifascist Fighters*]. VI Congrès Médical International de la F.I.R., Prague, 1976.

02640 DOBROWOLSKI, L.
Les Résultats des Examens Médicaux de Nombreux Groupes d'Anciens Prisonniers Hitleriens. [*Results of Medical Examinations of Some Groups of Former Hitler-Prisoners*]. VI Congrès Médical International de la F.I.R., Prague, 1976.

02650 DÖRING, G. K. Von
Spezifische Spätschäden Der Weiblichen Psyche Durch Die Politische Verfolgung. [*Specific Late Results of the Feminine Psyche through Political Persecution*]. In Paul, H. and H. J. Herberg (eds.), Psychische Spätschäden Nach Politischer Verfolgung. Basel: S. Karger, 1963, 155–168.

02660 DOMINIK, M.
Sytuacja Zdrowotna I Bytowa Bylych Wiezniow Oswiecimskich W Swietle Ankiety. [*The Health and Social Situation of Ex-Prisoners From Auschwitz*] (A Questionnaire Investigation). Przeglad Lekarski (1967) 24:102–104.

02670 DOMINIK, M.
Prisoners Respond to the Questionnaire. In Auschwitz, It Did Not End in Forty-Five, Anthology, Vol. 3, Part 1. Warsaw: International Auschwitz Committee, 1971.

02680 DOMINIK, M.; TEUTSCH, A.
Nerwice U Potostuwa Bylych Wiezniow Obozow Koncentracyjnych. [*Neuroses among the Children of Ex-Concentration Camp Prisoners*]. Przeglad Lekarski (1978) 35:16–20.

02690   DOMINIK, M.; TEUTSCH, A.
Neurosen Bei Der Nachkommenschaft Ehemaliger
Konzentrationslagerhäftlinge. [*Neuroses in the Offspring of Former
Concentration Camp Inmates*]. Mitteilungen Der F.I.R. (1978) 15:9–19.

02700   DOMINIK, M.
Potomstwo W Niektorych Rodzinach Bylych Wiezniow Hitlerowskich
Obozow Koncentracyjnych. [*The Children of Some Families of Former
Prisoners Of Hitlerian Concentration Camps*]. Przeglad Lekarski (1979)
36:25–38.

02710   DONNAY, J.M.; DETHIENNE, F.; MEYERS, C.
Incidence des Facteurs Traumatisants de la Captivitée sur la
Morbiditée Somatique et Psychiatrique de l'Ancien Prisonnier de
Guerre. [*The Incidence of Traumatizing Factors during Captivity on the
Somatic and Psychiatric Morbidity of Ex-Prisoners of War*]. Acta
Psychiat Belg (1975) 75:33–48.

02720   DORING, E.
Die Bedeutung Der Gesellschaftlichen Verhältnisse Für Eine Gunstige
Beeinflussung Der Häftspätschäden. [*The Meaning of Social Relations
for a Favourable Influence of the Sequelae of Imprisonment*]. In Cah
d'inf méd, soc jurid, (1983) 19:70–73.

02730   DOR-SHAV, N.K.
*On the Long-Range Effects of Concentration Camps on Nazi Victims
and Their Children.* Paper presented at the International Conference
on Psychological Stress and Adjustment in War and Peace, Tel Aviv,
1975.

02740   DOR-SHAV, N.K.
*On the Long-Range Effects of Concentration Camp Internment on Nazi
Victims: 25 Years Later.* J Consult and Clin Psychol (1978) 46(1):1–11.

02750   DOR-SHAV, N.K.
*Children of the Holocaust. A Study of the Second Generation of
Concentration Camp Survivors.* Manuscript.

02760   DREIFUSS, G.
The Analyst and the Damaged Victim of Nazi Persecution. J Anal
Psychol (1968) 14:163–175.

02770   DREIFUSS, G.
Psychotherapy of Nazi Victims. Psychother Psychosom (1980)
34:40–44.

02780   DREIFUSS, G.
Analysis of Holocaust Survivors. Paper presented at the Annual
Meeting of the International Association for Analytic Psychology, San
Francisco, September 1980. Manuscript.

02790   DREYFUS-MOREAU, J.
Etude Structurale de Deux Cas de Nevrose Concentrationnaire.
[*Structural Study of Two Cases of Neurosis in Concentration Camp
Inmates*]. Evolution Psychiat (1952) 1:201–220.

02800   DROHOCKI, Z.
Wstrzasy Elektryczne W Rewirze Monowickim. [*Electroshock
Treatment in the Monowitz Sick-Bay*]. Przeglad Lekarski (1975)
32:162–166.

02810   DUBIEL, A.
[*Recollections of a Sick Prisoner of the Neu Sustrum and Gusen
Concentration Camp*]. Przeglad Lekarski (1970) 26(1):216–219.

02820   DUNK, Von Der, H. W.
Some Remarks about the Consequences of World War II. In
Israel-Netherlands Symposium on the Impact of Persecution. 2,
Dalfsen, Amsterdam, 14–18 April 1980, The Netherlands: Rijswijk,
27–33.

02830   DVORJETSKI, M.
Biological and Pathological Problems of Camp Survivors in Israel. In
W.V.F. Experts Meeting on the Later Effects of Imprisonment and
Deportation, Oslo, 1960. Paris: World Veterans Federation, 1960,
89–97.

02840   DVORJETSKI, M.
*Biological and Sociological Problems of Camp Survivors Immigrants in
Israel.* In W.V.F. Experts Meeting on the Later Effects of
Imprisonment and Deportation. Oslo, 1960. Paris: World Veterans
Federation, 1960, 107–129.

02850   DVORJETSKI, M.
*Cardiac Pathology among Jewish Internees in Camps and Ghettos and
Cardiac Sequelae among Jewish Survivors.* [AB:12]. In Later Effects of
Imprisonment and Deportation. International Conference Organized
by the World Veterans Federation. The Hague: World Veterans
Federation, 1961, 39–52.

02860   DVORJETSKI, M.
*Integration into the Working Population and Vocational Rehabilitation
of Former Deportees in Israel.* In Later Effects of Imprisonment and
Deportation. International Conference Organized by the World
Veterans Federation. The Hague: World Veterans Federation, 1961,
150–157.

02870   DVORJETSKI, M.
Tuberculosis among Jewish Immigrants to Israel. In Later Effects of
Imprisonment and Deportation. International Conference Organized
by the World Veterans Federation. The Hague: World Veterans
Federation, 1961, 61–66.

02880   DYNER, E.
Specificité Multisyndromique des Maladies des Anciens Déportés.
[*The Multisyndrome Specificity of Diseases in Formerly Deported
Persons*]. VI Congrès Médical International de la F.I.R., Prague, 1976.

02890   DYNER, E.; GLOWACKI, C.
Evaluation de l'état de Santé Actuel des Anciens Déportés, Faite sur
la Base des Examens Médicaux Poursuivis dans Plusieurs Milieux de

Varsovie. [*Evaluation of the Present State of Health of Former Deportees on the Basis of Medical Follow-Up Examinations in Several Districts of Warsaw*]. VI Congrès Médical International de la F.I.R., Prague, 1976.

02900   DZIADU'S, S.
[*"Hirschberg" and "Treskau" Branches of the Gross-Rosen Concentration Camp. Excerpts from the Memoirs*]. Przeglad Lekarski (1969) 25(1):138–145.

02910   DZIADU'S, S.
[*The Penal Company at the Gross-Rosen Concentration Camp*]. Przeglad Lekarski (1970) 26(1):223–228.

02930   DZIADU'S, S.
[*The Saurer-Werke Camp after Liberation*]. Przeglad Lekarski (1975) 32(1):178–82.

02940   EATON, W.W.; SIGAL, J.J.; WEINFELD, M.
Impairment in Holocaust Survivors after 33 Years: Data from an Unbiased Community Sample. Am J Psychiat (1982) 139:773–777.

02950   ECKSTAEDT, A.
Eine Klinische Studie Zum Begriff Der Traumareaktion, Ein Kindheitsschicksal Aus Der Kriegszeit. [*A Clinical Study for the Understanding of the Traumatic Reaction, A Child's Fate as a Consequence of the War*]. Psyche (1981) 35(7):600–610.

02960   EDEL, E.
Kausalitätsnachweis Bei Begutachtung Von Gesundheitsschäden Infolge Politischer Verfolgung. [*Probing Causality in the Evaluation of Health Damage as a Result of Political Persecution*]. In Ermüdung Und Vorzeitiges Altern. Folge Von Extremebelastungen. V Internationaler Medizinischer Kongress Der F.I.R., Paris, 1970. Leipzig: Johann Ambrosius, 1973, 308–314.

02970   EDEL, E.
Zur Problematik Der Behandlungsfähigkeit Der Zweiten Generation. [*On the Problems of Treatment Possibility in the Second Generation*]. VI Internationaler Medizinischer Kongress Der F.I.R., Prague, 1976.

02980   EDELSTEIN, E. L.
Reactivation of Concentration Camp Experiences as a Result of Hospitalization. In Milgram, N. (ed.), Stress and Anxiety. Washington: Hemisphere Publishing, 1982, 401–404.

02990   EISSLER, K.R.
Variationen In Der Psychoanalytischen Technique. [*Variations in Psychoanalytic Technique*]. Psyche (1960) 13:609–624.

03000   EISSLER, K.R.
Die Ermordung Von Wievielen Seiner Kinder Muss Ein Mensch Symptomfrei Ertragen Können, Um Eine Normale Konstitution Zu Haben? [*The Murder of How Many of His Children Must a Person Be Able to Endure Symptomless in Order to Have a Normal Constitution?*]. Psyche (1963) 17:241–291.

03010   EISSLER, K.R.
Pervertierte Psychiatrie? [*Perverted Psychiatry?*]. Psyche (1967)
8:533–575. Also in Am J Psychiat (1967) 123:1352–1358.

03020   EISSLER, K.R.
Wietere Bemerkungen Zum Problem Der KZ Psychologie. Diskussion
Des Vortrages Von Dr. E. De Wind. [*Additional Comments to the
Problem of the Concentration Camp Psychology. Discussion of Dr.
E. De Wind's Lecture*]. Psyche (1968) 22:452–463.

03025   EITINGER, L.
Sykehus behandlingen i Konsentrasjons leiren Auschwitz. [*Hospital
Treatment in Auschwitz Concentration Camp*]. Tidsskr Norske
Lageforen (1945) 65:159–161.

03030   EITINGER, L.
The Symptomatology of Mental Disease among Refugees in Norway. J
Ment Sci (1960) 106:947–966.

03040   EITINGER, L.
Psychiatric Delayed Effects of Internment in Concentration Camps. In
W.V.F. Experts Meeting on the Late Effects of Imprisonment and
Deportation, Oslo, 1960, 55–66.

03050   EITINGER, L.
Psykiatriske Folgetilstander Hos Tidligere Konsentrasjonsleirfanger.
[*Psychiatric Sequelae in Concentration Camp Ex-Prisoners*]. In
Strøm, A., Undersokelse Av Norske Tidligere
Konsentrasjonsleirfanger (1961) 81:805–808.

03060   EITINGER, L.
Pathology of the Concentration Camp Syndrome. Arch Gen Psychiat
(1961) 5:371–379.

03070   EITINGER, L.
Psychiatric Post Conditions in Former Concentration Camp Inmates. In
Later Effects of Imprisonment and Deportation. International
Conference Organized by the World Veterans Federation. The Hague:
World Veterans Federation, 1961.

03080   EITINGER, L.
Concentration Camp Survivors in the Postwar World. Am J
Orthopsychiat (1962) 32:367–375.

03090   EITINGER, L.
Refugees and Concentration Camp Survivors in Norway. Isr Med J
(1962) 21(1–2):21–27.

03100   EITINGER, L.
*Preliminary Notes on a Study of Concentration Camp Survivors in
Norway*. Isr Ann Psychiat and Rel Disc (1963) 1:59–67.

03110   EITINGER, L.
Schizophrenia and Persecution. Acta Psychiat Scand (1964)
40(180):141–146. Rev. in the Author's Book, Concentration Camp
Survivors in Norway and Israel, 1964.

03120   EITINGER, L.
Tidligere Konsentrasjonsleirfanger I Norge Og I Israel. [*Former Concentration Camp Inmates in Norway and Israel*]. Nordisk Med (1964) 72:1207–1212.

03130   EITINGER, L.
Concentration Camp Survivors in Norway and Israel. The Hague: Martinus Nijhoff, 1972. First published by the Norwegian Research Council for Science and Humanities, 1964.

03140   EITINGER, L.
Der Parrallelismus Zwischen Dem KZ Syndrom Und Der Chronischen Anorexia Nervosa. [*The Parallelism of the Concentration Camp Syndrome and Chronic Anorexia Nervosa*]. Anorexia Nervosa. Symposium Ed: Meyer, J. E. Und H. Georg Thieme Feldmann. Stuttgart, 1965, 118–122.

03150   EITINGER, L.
Concentration Camp Survivors in Norway and Israel. In David, H. P. (ed.), Migration, Mental Health and Community Services. Geneva: American Joint Distribution Committee, 1966, 14–22.

03160   EITINGER, L.
The Late Effects of Chronic Excessive Stress on Two Different Population Groups. Excerpta Medica International Congress No. 150, Proceedings of the IV World Congress of Psychiatry, Madrid, 1966, 912–917.

03170   EITINGER, L.
Schizophrenia among Concentration Camp Survivors. Int J Psychiat (1967) 3:403–406.

03180   EITINGER, L.; ASKEVOLD, F.
Psychiatric Aspects. In Strøm, A. (ed.), Norwegian Concentration Camp Survivors. Oslo: Universitetsforlaget; New York: Humanities Press, 1968, 45–84.

03190   EITINGER, L.
Attforingsproblemer Hos Tidliger Konsentrasjonsleirfanger. [*Rehabilitation Problems in Ex-Prisoners*]. Samtiden (1968) 53:518–525.

03200   EITINGER, L.
Rehabilitation of Concentration Camp Survivors (Following Concentration Camp Trauma). Psychother and Psychosom (1969) 17:42–49.

03210   EITINGER, L.
Psychosomatic Problems in Concentration Camp Survivors. J Psychosom Res (1969) 13:183–189.

03220   EITINGER, L.
Anxiety in Concentration Camp Survivors. Austral NZ J Psychiat (1969) 3:348–351.

03230   EITINGER, L.
Syndrom Koncentracnich Taboru. (Byvali Norsti Vezni Nemeckych
Koncentracnich Taboru). [*The Concentration Camp
Syndrome—Former Norwegian Concentration Camp Prisoners*].
Ceskoslovenska Psychiat (1970) 66:257–266.

03240   EITINGER, L.
*Organic and Psychosomatic Aftereffects of Concentration Camp
Imprisonment*. In Krystal, H. and W. Niederland (eds.), Massive
Traumatization. Boston: Little, Brown, 1970, 205–215.

03250   EITINGER, L.
Psychiatrische Untersuchungsergebnisse Bei KZ-Ueberlebenden.
[*Results of Psychiatric Examinations in Survivors of Concentration
Camps*]. In Herberg, H. J. (ed.), Spätschäden Nach
Extremebelastungen. II Internationalen Medizinisch-Juristischen
Konferenz in Düsseldorf, 1969. Herford: Nicolaische
Verlagsbuchhandlung, 1971, 144–152.

03260   EITINGER, L.
Newer Investigations on Concentration Camp Survivors. Anali Bolnice
Dr. Stojanovic, M. (1971) 10:201–206.

03270   EITINGER, L.
*Acute and Chronic Psychiatric and Psychosomatic Reactions in
Concentration Camp Survivors*. In Levi, Lennart, Society, Stress and
Disease. New York: Oxford University Press, 1971, 219–230.

03280   EITINGER, L.
Umrtnost A Nemocnost Po Excesivnim Stressu. [*Mortality and
Morbidity after Excessive Stress*]. Ceskoslovenska Psychiat (1973)
69:209–218.

03290   EITINGER, L.; STRØM, A.
Mortality and Morbidity after Excessive Stress. Oslo:
Universitetsforlaget; New York: Humanities Press, 1973.

03300   EITINGER, L.
*Late Effects of Imprisonment in Concentration Camps during World
War II*. In Phsysical and Mental Consequences of Imprisonment and
Torture. Lectures presented at the Conference at Lysebu near Oslo,
1973. London: Amnesty International, 1973, 90–113.

03310   EITINGER, L.
*A Follow-Up Study of the Norwegian Concentration Camp Survivors'
Mortality and Morbidity*. Isr Ann Psychiat and Rel Disc (1973)
11(3):199–209.

03320   EITINGER, L.
Coping with Aggression. Ment Health and Soc (1974) 1:297–301.

03330   EITINGER, L.
Jewish Concentration Camp Survivors in Norway. Isr Ann Psychiat and
Rel Disc (1975) 13(4):321–334.

03340   EITINGER, L.
Stress and Personality. VI Congrès Médical International de la F.I.R.,
Prague, 1976.

03350   EITINGER, L.
On Being a Psychiatrist and a Survivor. Rosenfeld, A. H. and
I. Greenberg, (eds.), Confronting the Holocaust. London: Indiana
University Press, 1978, 186–230.

03360   EITINGER, L.
Psychological and Psychiatric Aftereffects of the Holocaust. Conference
on the Aftermath of the Holocaust, Haifa, 1979. Manuscript.

03370   EITINGER, L.
Report on Establishing a Reprint Library and Bibliography on
Concentration Camp Survivors. Presentation at meeting in Tel-Aviv,
1979. Manuscript.

03380   EITINGER, L.
Transcultural Literature on Second Generation. First International
Conference on Children of Survivors, New York, 1979. Manuscript.

03390   EITINGER, L.
Jewish Concentration Camp Survivors in the Post-War World. Danish
Med Bull (1980) 27(5):224–228.

03400   EITINGER, L.
The Concentration Camp Syndrome and Its Late Sequelae. In Dimsdale,
J. E. (ed.), Survivors, Victims and Perpetrators. Washington:
Hemisphere Publishing, 1980, 127–160.

03410   EITINGER, L.
Studies on Concentration Camp Survivors: The Norwegian and Global
Contexts. J Psychol Judaism (1981) 6:23–32.

03420   EITINGER, L.; RIECK, M.
Bibliographical Collection of Literature Concerning Medical and
Psychological Sequelae to Concentration Camp Imprisonment. Ray
D. Wolfe Centre for Study of Psychological Stress, Haifa University,
1981. Theoretical Introduction to Computerized Comprehensive
Bibliographical List. Manuscript.

03430   EITINGER, L.; STRØM, A.
New Investigations on the Mortality and Morbidity of Norwegian
Ex-Concentration Camp Prisoners. Isr J Psychiat Rel Sci (1981)
18:173–195.

03440   EITINGER, L.
Denial in Concentration Camps. Nord Psykiatr Tidsskr (1981)
5:148–156.

03450   EITINGER, L.
Den Medicinsk-Psykiatrske Litteraturen Om "Spatschaden." [The
Medical-Psychiatric Literature on Compensation]. Nordisk
Judaistik-Scandinavian Jewish Studies (1982) 4:2–10.

03460 EITINGER, L.
Jewish Concentration Camp Survivors. In Ayalon, O. (ed.), The Holocaust and Its Perseverance. Assen, Holland, 1983, 4– 16.

03470 ELIASBERG, W. G.
Theory and Practice in the Psychiatric Evaluation of Restitution Cases. Isr Ann Psychiat (1964) 2:81– 92.

03480 ELIASBERG, W. G.
Older and Recent Psychiatric Views on the Victims of Nazi Persecution. Harefuah (1967) 72:347– 348.

03490 ELLENBOGEN, R.
Frequency and Gravity of the Various Diseases and Disabilities among Survivors of Concentration Camps. In Later Effects of Imprisonment and Deportation. International Conference Organized by the World Veterans Federation. The Hague: World Veterans Federation, 1961, 115– 121.

03500 ELLENBOGEN, R.
Die Beurteilung Der Folgen Von Internierung Und Deportation In Frankreich. [*The Evaluation of the Sequels of Internment and Deportation in France*]. In Herberg, H.J. (ed.), Beurteilung von Gesundheitsschäden Nach Gefangenschaft Und Verfolgung. Internationalen Medizinische-Juristischen Symposiums in Köln (1967). Herford: Nicolaische Verlagsbuchhandlung, 1967. 34– 43.

03510 ELZAS, J.
Prognoses van de in 1926 en later geboren vervolgden. [*Prognoses of the Persecuted Born in 1926 and Later*]. Jerusalem, 1976. Manuscript.

03520 ELZAS, J.
Persecution and Its Effects. Jerusalem, 1977. Manuscript.

03530 ENGEL, W. H.
Reflections on the Psychiatric Consequences of Persecution. An Evaluation of Restitution Claimants. Am J Psychother (1962) 16:191– 203.

03550 ENGELS, D. E.
Uit naam van, een literatuurstudie naar de kinderen van overlevenden van de tweede wereldoorlog. [*In the Name of, A Study of the Literature of Children of Survivors of the Second World War*]. Ph.D. diss., 1982. U. of Groningen.

03560 ENGELS, D. E.
Het postconcentratiekampsyndroom. [*The Post Concentration Camp Syndrome*]. Tijdschr Psychother (1983) 9(5):215– 229.

03570 ENGESET, A.
Luftencefalografiske Funn Hos Tidligere Konsentrasjonsleirfanger. [*Pneumoencephalographic Findings in Ex-Prisoners*]. Tidsskr Norske Loegeforering (1961) 81:810– 811.

03580 ENGESET, A.
Pneumoencephalographic Findings in Ex-Concentration Camp Inmates.

In Later Effects of Imprisonment and Deportation. International Conference Organized by the World Veterans Federation. The Hague: World Veterans Federation, 1961, 93– 95.

03590   ENGESET, A.
Pneumoencephalographical Examinations. In Strøm, A. (ed.), Norwegian Concentration Camp Survivors. Oslo: Universitetsforlaget; New York: Humanities Press, 1968, 124– 131.

03600   EPSTEIN, A. W.
Mental Phenomena across Generations: The Holocaust. J Am Acad Psychoanal (1982) 10(4):565– 570.

03610   EPSTEIN, B. B.
Meeting in Tel-Aviv. In Steinitz, L. (ed.), Living after the Holocaust: Reflections by the Post-War Generation in America. New York: Bloch, 1975, 93– 100.

03620   EPSTEIN, H.
Children of the Holocaust: Conversations with Sons and Daughters of Survivors. New York: Putnam, 1979.

03630   FABOWSKA-GRZEZULKO, Z.
[Evacuation From the Ravensbruck-Wattenstedt Concentration Camp]. Przeglad Lekarski (1977) 34(1):198– 200.

03640   FALGOWSKI, J.
[Health Facilities Provided by the SS at the Majdanek Concentration Camp]. Przeglad Lekarski (1970) 26(1):172– 3.

03650   FALEK, A.; BRITTON, S.
Phases in Coping: The Hypothesis and Its Implications. Soc Biol 21 (1):1– 7.

03660   FAUST, C.
Hirnatrophie Nach Hungerdystrophie. *[Atrophy of the Brain after Malnutrition].* Nervenarzt (1952) 23:406.

03670   FAUST, C.
[Chronic Reactive Depression. Disorders Following Imprisonment and Persecution]. Fortschr Med (1983) 10;101(9):372– 376.

03680   FEDERN, E.
Terror as a System: The Concentration Camp. Buchenwald As It Was. Psychiatr Q, Suppl (1948) 22:52, Part 1.

03690   FEDERN, E.
The Endurance of Torture. Complex (1951) 4:34– 41.

03700   FEDERN, E.
Some Clinical Remarks on the Psychopathology of Genocide. Psychiat Q (1960) 34:538– 549.

03710   FEDEROWICZ, T.
[Attitude of the Concentration Camp Physicians]. Przeglad Lekarski (1970) 26(1):238– 242.

03720   FEJKIEL, W.
Typhus Exantematicus at Oswiecim Concentration Camp from 1941–1945. Rozpr Wydz Manknud (1958) 3:5–50.

03730   FEJKIEL, W.
Health Service in the Auschwitz I Concentration Camp, Main Camp. In Auschwitz, In Hell They Preserved Human Dignity, Anthology, Vol. 2, Part 1. Warsaw: International Auschwitz Committee, 1971, 4–37.

03740   FEJKIEL, W.
Bewertung Des Gesundheitszustandes Ehemaliger Auschwitz-Häftlinge An Denen Verbrecherische Experimente Vorgenommen Worden Sino. [*Evaluation of the State of Health of Former Auschwitz Prisoners, Who Underwent Criminal Experimentation*]. In Ermüdung Und Vorzeitiges Altern. Folge Von Extremebelastungen. V Internationaler Medizinischer Kongress Der F.I.R., Paris, 1970. Leipzig: Johann Ambrosius, 1973, 315–320.

03750   FEJKIEL, W.
[*Lasting Defects and Changes in the System Following Epidemic Typhus (Author's Translation)*]. Przeglad Lekarski (1975) 32(8):668–671.

03760   FEJKIEL, W.
Dauerschäden Und Pathologische Veränderungen Im Organismus Als Folge Des Fleckfiebers. [*Permanent Damage and Pathological Modifications in the Organism as Sequelae of Typhus*]. VI Internationaler Medizinischer Kongress Der F.I.R., Prague, 1976.

03770   FEJKIEL, W.
Das Infektionskrankheitsbild Und Dessen Epidemien In Künstlich Gebildeter Gemeinschaft In Konzentrations Lager Auschwitz. [*The Infections Disease Syndrome and its Epidemics in Artificially Created Groups in the Concentration Camp Auschwitz*]. VI Internationaler Medizinischer Kongress Der F.I.R., Prague, 1976.

03780   FEUERSTEIN, C. W.
Working with the Holocaust Victims Psychologically. J Contemp Psychother (1980) 11:70–77.

03790   FICHEZ, L. F.
Die Chronische Progressive Asthenie. Materialien Der Internationalen Konferenzen Von Kopenhagen Und Miskau, Zusammengestellt Vom Ärztlichen Sekretariat Der Internationalen Föderation Der Widerstandskämpfer. (1958). [*The Chronic Progessive Asthenia*]. Miskau: Verlag Der F.I.R., n.d., Band 2.

03800   FICHEZ, L. F.
Andere Spätfolgen. Medizinische Konferenzen Der Internationalen Federation Der Widerstandkämpfer Von Kopenhagen Und Miskau. [*Other Late Sequelae*]. Austria: Verlag Der F.I.R., 1959, Band 2. Papers by: Gukassian, Gilbert, Dreyfus, Franck, Sterboul, Heller, Reicl, Worms, Desoille, Deveen, Wetterwald, Fichez, and Weinstein.

03810   FICHEZ, L. F.; WEINSTEIN, S.
Die Tuberkulose Bei Den Französischen Überlebenden Der

Nazistischen Gefängnisse Und Vernichtungslager. [*Tuberculosis in French Survivors of the Nazi Prisons and Extermination Camps*]. In Fichez, L. (ed.), Andere Spätfolgen. Austria: Verlag Der F.I.R., 1959, Band 2, 77–88.

03820   FICHEZ, L. F.; KLOTZ, A.
Die Vorzeitige Vergreisung Und Ihre Behandlung An Hand Von Beobachtungen An Ehemaligen Deportierten Und KZ-Häftlingen. [*Premature Aging and Its Treatment According to the Observations of Former Deportees and Concentration Camp Prisoners*]. Vienna: Verlag Der F.I.R., 1961.

03830   FICHEZ, L. F.; LANDAU, A.
Schlaftherapie Bei Chronischer Asthenie Und Vorzeitiger Seneszenz Ehemaliger Deportierter Und Konzentrationslagerinsassen. [*Sleep Therapy of Chronic Asthenia and Premature Aging in Former Deportees and Concentration Camp Inmates*]. In Ätio-Pathogenese Und Therapie Der Erschöpfung Und Vorzeitigen Veargreisung. IV Internationaler Medizinischer Kongress Der F.I.R. Bucharest: Verlag Der F.I.R., 1964, 421–426.

03840   FICHEZ, L. F.
L'Etio-Pathogénie et la Thérapeutique de l'Asthenie et de la Senescence Premature. [*The Etio-Pathology and the Treatment of Asthenia and Premature Aging*]. Bucharest, 1964.

03850   FICHEZ, L. F.
Eröffnungsansprach. [*Opening Speech*]. Ermüdung Und Vorzeitiges Altern. Folge von Extremebelastungen. V Internationaler Medizinischer Kongress Der F.I.R., Paris, 1970. Leipzig: Johann Ambrosius, 1973, 20–25.

03860   FICHEZ, L. F.
Stoffwechselstörungen Als Folge Des Hungers Und Psycho-Physiologische Probleme Der Ermüdung Und Vorzeitigen Vergreisung. [*Metabolic Disturbances as a Result of Hunger and Psycho-Physiological Problems of Fatigue and Premature Aging*]. Mitteilungen Der F.I.R. (1975) 9:1–9.

03870   FICHEZ, L. F.
Etude de morbidité à long terme chez les anciens deportés des camps d'extermination nazis. [*Study of the Long Term Morbidity of Former Deportees from Nazi Extermination Camps*]. In Cah d'inf méd soc jurid (1983) 19:104–116.

03880   FICHEZ, L. F.
Premiers résultats de l'étude du bilan lipidique des anciens deportés hommes et femmes hospitalisés dans un centre specialisé. [*First Results of the Study of the Lipid Balance of Former Deported Men and Women Hospitalized in a Specialized Centre*]. In Cah d'inf méd, soc jurid (1983) 19:117–121.

03890   FINK, H. F.
Development Arrest as a Result of Nazi Persecution During Adolescence. . Int J Psycho-Anal (1968) 49(2–3):327–329.

03900   FINK, K. P.
        Victims of Political-Racial Persecution. Nurs Times (1979)
        75(12):496–499.

03910   FISCHER, O.
        Die Bedeutung Der Amoebenruhr Als Versorgungs Und
        Verfolgungsleiden. [*The Importance of Amoebic Dysentery as a Disease
        Caused by Persecution and Entitled for Compensation*]. In Herberg,
        H. J. (ed.), Die Beurteilung Von Gesundheitsschäden Nach
        Gefangenschaft Und Verfolgung. Internationalen
        Medizinisch-Juristischen Symposiums in Köln (1967). Herford:
        Nicolaische Verlagsbuchhandling, 1967, 102–107.

03920   FISHBANE, M. D.
        Children of Survivors of the Nazi Holocaust: A Psychological Inquiry.
        Ph.D. diss., University of Massachusetts, 1979. Page 449 in Vol.
        40/01-B of Dissertation Abstracts International. Order No:
        AAD79-12680.

03930   FISHER S. H.
        Psychiatric Symptomatology and Later Effects in War Imprisonment. In
        Experts Meeting on the Later Effects of Imprisonment and
        Deportation. Oslo, 1960. Paris: World Veterans Federation, 1960,
        67–78.

03940   FITZEK, J. M.; HERBERG, H. J.
        Auslesegesichtspunkte Und Allgemeine Erfahrungen Bei Den
        Untersuchungen Des Köllner Arbeitskreises. [*Points of View in
        Selection and General Experiences of the Investigations Done by the
        Working Group of Cologne*]. In Paul, H. and H. J. Herberg (eds.),
        Psychische Spätsschäden Nach Politischer Verfolgung. Basel:
        S. Karger, 1963, 169–178.

03950   FLOUNTZIS, A.
        Besonderheiten Des Problems Der Asthenie Und Des Vorzeitigen
        Alterns Der Grieschischen Antifaschistischen Deportierten Und
        Häftlinge. [*Peculiarities of the Problem of Asthenia and Premature
        Ageing of Greek Antifascist Deportees and Prisoners*]. In
        Aetio-Pathogenese Und Therapie Der Erschoepfung Und Vorzeitigen
        Vergreisung. IV Internationaler Medizinischer Kongress Der F.I.R.
        Bucharest: Verlag Der F.I.R., 1964, 337–343.

03960   FODOR, R.
        *The Impact of Nazi Occupation of Poland on the Jewish Mother-Child
        Relationship.* YIVO Annual of Jewish Social Sciences (1956/57) v.11.

03970   FOGELMAN, E.; SAVRAN, B.
        Therapeutic Groups for Children of Holocaust Survivors. Am J
        Orthopsychiat (1979) 29:211–235.

03980   FOGELMAN, E.; SAVRAN, B.
        Therapeutic Groups with Children of Holocaust Survivors. Int J Group
        Psychother (1979) 29(2):211–236.

03990   FOGELMAN, E.
*Brief Group Therapy with Offspring of Holocaust Survivors: Leaders'
Reactions.* Am J Orthopsychiat (1980) 50(1):96–108.

04000   FORBERT, A.
[*In Auschwitz after Liberation*]. Przeglad Lekarski (1980)
37(1):182–184.

04010   FRACKOWSKI, K.
[*Jews and Priests at the Sachsenhausen-Orianienburg Concentration
Camp*]. Przeglad Lekarski (1970) 26(1):159–164.

04020   FRANASZEK, E.; CHLEBOWSKA, M.; HOEHNE, T.
Stan Jamy Ustnej Wiezniow W Obozach Koncentracyjnych (W
Swietle Badan Ankietowich). [*The Oral and Dental Status in the
Concentration Camps (A Questionnaire Investigation)*]. Przeglad
Lekarski (1977) 34:25–28.

04030   FRANCI'C, V.
[*An Organization of University Professors, Inmates of the
Sachsenhausen Concentration Camp*]. Przeglad Lekarski (1970)
26(1):150–158.

04040   FRANKEL, H.
The Survivor as a Parent. J Jewish Communal Serv (1978)
54(3):241–246.

04050   FRANKL, V. E.
Group Therapeutic Experiences in a Concentration Camp. Group
Psychother (1954) 7:81–90.

04060   FRANKL, V. E.
*From Death Camp to Existentialism, A Psychiatrist's Path to a New
Therapy.* Boston: Beacon Press, 1959.

04070   FRANKL, V. E.
Psychologie Und Psychiatrie Des Konzentrationslagers. [*The
Psychology and Psychiatry of the Concentration Camps*]. In Psychiatrie
Der Gegenwart. Berlin, Göttingen, Heidelberg: Springer Verlag, 1961,
743–759.

04080   FRANKL, V. E.
On the Psychology of the Concentration Camp. In The Doctor and the
Soul. New York: Knopf, 1965. 93–104.

04090   FRANKL, V. E.
Higiena Psychiczna W Sytuacji Przymusowej Doswiadczenia Z
Zakresu Psychoterapii W Obozie Koncentracyjnym. [*Mental Hygiene
in an Extreme Situation: A Psychotherapeutic Experience From the
Concentration Camp*]. In Piaty Zeszyt Poswiecony Zagdnieniom
Lekarskim Okresu Hitlerowskiej Okupdciji. Przeglad Lekarski (1965)
21(1):24–28.

04100   FRANKL, V. E.
... Trotzdem Ja Zum Leben Sagen. Ein Psychologe Erlebt Das

Konsentrationslager Sage. [*Life Has Meaning (Say Yes to Life, In Spite of Everything...) A Psychologist in the Concentration Camp*]. München: Kösel-Verlag, 1979.

04110   FRANKL, V. E.
Man's Search for Meaning. An Introduction to Logotherapy. Boston: Beacon Press, 1962.

04120   FRENK, S.
[*Non Omnis Moriar. Forty Years after the Clinical Research on Hunger Performed in 1942 in the Warsaw Ghetto*]. Gac Med Mex (1982) 118(12):509–513.

04130   FREUD, A.; DANN, S.
An Experiment in Group Upbringing. Psychoanal Study of the Child. New York: Internat. Universities Press (1951) 6:127–141.

04140   FRESCO, N.
La Diaspora des Cendres. [*The Diaspora of the Ashes*]. Nouvelle Revue de Psychanalyse (1981) 24:205–220.

04150   FREYBERG, J.T.
Difficulties in Separation-Individuation As Experienced by Offspring of Nazi Holocaust Survivors. Am J Orthopsychiat (1980) 50:87–95.

04160   FREYBERGER, H.; HERTZ, D.G.
Experiences in Dealing with the Evaluations of the Former Nazi Persecuted: Now Living in Israel, South America, North America and Canada. Manuscript.

04170   FRIEDMAN, P.
The Effects of Imprisonment. Acta Med Orientalia (1948) 7:163–167.

04180   FRIEDMAN, P.
The Road Back for the D.P.s: Healing the Psychological Scars of Nazism. Commentary (1948) 6:502–510.

04190   FRIEDMAN, P.
Some Aspects of Concentration Camp Psychology. Am J Psychiat (1949) 105:601–605.

04200   FULLY, G.
Abhandlung Über Die Pathogenese Der Wirbelschäden Aufgrund Anatomischer Festellungen, Die An Skeletten Von Deportierten, Welche in Den Deutschen Konzentrationslagern Verstorben Sind, Gemacht Wurden. [*Report about the Pathogenesis of Damage to the Vertebrae, Based on Anatomical Findings, Which Were Established on the Skeletons of Those Who Died in German Concentration Camps*]. In Aetio-Pathogenese Und Therapie Der Erschöpfung Und Vorzeitigen Vergreisung. IV Internationaler Medizinischer Kongress Der F.I.R. Bucharest: Verlag Der F.I.R., 1964, 291–295.

04210   FURMAN, E.
The Impact of the Nazi Concentration Camps on the Children of Survivors. In Anthony, E.J. and C. Koupernik (eds.), The Child in His

Family: The Impact of Disease and Death. New York: Wiley, 1973, 379–384.

04230   GAMPEL, Y.
A Daughter of Silence. In Bergmann, M. S. and M. E. Jucovy (eds.), Generations of the Holocaust. New York: Basic Books, 1982, 120–136.

04240   GARLAND, C.
(Ed.). *The Survivor Syndrome Workshop*. Group Analysis Journal, November 1980. Special Issue. With papers by Lifton, Davidson, and Herman and reports from group discussions.

04250   GARMADA, L.
[*Reminiscences from the Janow Concentration Camp*]. Przeglad Lekarski (1978) 35(1):166–170.

04260   GARSTKA, S. M.
[*The Nazi Concentration Camp in Flossenberg*]. Przeglad Lekarski (1974) 31(1):191–195.

04270   GARTLAND, P. A. F.
Out of the Burning: Response to the Holocaust. Ph.D. diss., University of Iowa, 1981. Page 3155 in Vol. 42/07-A of Dissertation Abstracts International. Order No: AAD81-28391.

04280   GATARSKI, J.
Badania Elektroencefalograficzne U Osob Urodzonych Lub Przebywajacych W Dziecinstwie W Hitlerowskich Obozach Koncentracyjnych. [*Electroencephalographic Findings in Persons Who Either Were Born in Concentration Camps or Spent Their Earlier Life There*]. Przeglad Lekarski (1966) 23:37–38.

04290   GATARSKI, J.
Electroencephalographic Examinations of People Born in Camps or Who Had Stayed in Their Childhood in Nazi Concentration Camps. In Auschwitz, In Hell They Preserved Human Dignity, Anthology, Vol. 2, Part 3. Warsaw: International Auschwitz Committee, 1971, 133–142.

04300   GATARSKI, J.; DRWID, M.; MALGORZATA, D.
Wyniki Badania Psychiatryczego I Elektroencefalograficznego 130 Bylych Wiezniow Oswiecimia-Brzezinki. [*Results of Psychiatric and Electroencephalographic Investigations of Ex-Prisoners from Auschwitz-Birkenau*]. Przeglad Lekarski (1978) 35:29–32.

04310   GAWALEWICZ, A.
Waiting Room for the Gas. In Auschwitz, Anthology, Vol. 2, Part 1. Warsaw: International Auschwitz Committee, 1971, 107–149.

04320   GAWALEWICZ, A.
A Number Gets Back Its Name. In Auschwitz, Anthology Vol. 3, Part 1. Warsaw: International Auschwitz Committee, 1971, 4–66.

04330   GAWALEWICZ, J.; JACEQICZ, W.
Wymieralnosc W Latach 1945–1976 Bylych Wiezniow Dachau, Duchownych Rzymskokatolickich. [*The Mortality during the Years*

1945–1976 of Roman Catholic Priests Who Have Been Prisoners in Dachau]. Przeglad Lekarski (1978) 35:29–32.

04340　GAWRYLUK, F.
[Reminiscences from the Flossenburg Camp]. Przeglad Lekarski (1975) 35(1):171–178.

04350　GAY, M.
Children of Ex-Concentration Camp Inmates. In Miller, L. (ed.), Mental Health in Rapid Social Change. Jerusalem: Academic Press, 1972, 337–338.

04360　GAY, M.; FUCHS, J.; BLITTNER, M.
Characteristics of the Offspring of Holocaust Survivors in Israel. Ment Health Soc (1974) 1:302–312.

04370　GAY, M.; SHULMAN, S.
Comparison of Children of Holocaust Survivors with Children of the General Population of Israel: Are Children of Holocaust-Survivor Parents More Disturbed Than Others? Ment Health Soc (1978) 5(5–6):252–256.

04380　GAY, M.
The Adjustment of Parents to Wartime Bereavement. In Milgram, N. (ed.), Stress and Anxiety. Washington: Hemisphere Publishing, 1982, 243–247.

04390　GILBERT-DREYFUSS, H.; FICHEZ, L.F.; FRANCK, L.J.
Guenstige Wirkungen Der Schlafkur Bei Ehemaligen Deportierten Mit Asthenischer Abmagerung Auch Zusammen Mit Lungentuberkulose. *[Beneficial Effects of Sleep Therapy with Former Deportees Being Asthenically Thin, Also with Lung Tuberculosis]*. In Michel, M. (ed.), Gesundheitsschäden Durch Verfolgung Und Gefangenschaft Und Irhe Spätfolgen. Frankfurt Am Main: Röderberg Verlag, 1955, 317–323. Also in Fichez, L.F. (ed.), Andere Spätfolgen. Medizinisch Konferenzen Der Internationalen Federation Der Widerstandkämpfer Von Kopenhagen Und Miskau. Austria: Verlag Der F.I.R., 1959, Band 2, 52–63.

04400　GILBERT-DREYFUSS, H.; FRANCK, L.J.
Die Ernährungsstörungen Bei Den Deportierten. *[Nutritional Disturbances in Deportees]*. In Michel, M. (ed.), Gesundheitsschäden Durch Verfolgung Und Gefangenschaft Und Ihre Spätfolgen. Frankfurt Am Main: Roederberg Verlag, 1955, 107–126. Also in Fichez, L.F. (ed.), Andere Spätfolgen. Medizinisch Konferenzen Der Internationalen Federation Der Widerstandkämpfer Von Kopenhagen Und Miskau. Austria: Verlag Der F.I.R., 1959, Band 2, 25–32.

04410　GILBERT-DREYFUSS, H.
Die Funktionelle Nebennierenschwäche Der Ehemaligen Häftlinge. *[The Functional Weakness of the Adrenals in Former Internees]*. In Fichez, L.F. (ed.), Andere Spätfolgen. Austria: Verlag Der F.I.R., 1959, Band 2, 33–40.

04420   GILBERT-DREYFUSS, H.; SEBAOUN, J.; ZARA, M.
Thyroid Disorders Following Concentration Camp Internment. In Later
Effects of Imprisonment and Deportation. International Conference
Organized by the World Veterans Federation. The Hague: World
Veterans Federation, 1961, 69–72.

04430   GIZA, J.S.; MORASIEWICZ, W.
[*Problem of Impulsiveness in Concentration Camps. Analysis of the
Concentration Camp Syndrome*]. Przeglad Lekarski (1973) 30(1):29–41.

04440   GIZA, J.S.; MORASIEWICZ, W.
Poobozowe Zaburzenia Seksualne U Kobiet Jako Element Tzw KZ
Syndromu. [*Post Concentration Camp Sexual Disturbances among
Women as an Element of the So-Called Concentration Camp Syndrome*].
Przeglad Lekarski (1974) 31:65–75.

04450   GIZA, J.S.
Die Lager Problematik In Den Untersuchungen Amerikanischer
Psychiater. [*The Problems of the Camp in the Examinations by
American Psychiatrists*]. Mitteilungen Der F.I.R. (1975) 9:15–20.

04460   GIZA, J.S.
Problematyka Obozowa W Badaniach Psychiatrow Amery Kanskich.
[*Concentration Camp Problems Studied by American Psychiatrists*].
Przeglad Lekarski (1975) 32(1):209–211.

04470   GLICKSMAN, W.
Social Differentiation in the German Concentration Camps. In
Fishman, J.A. (ed.), Studies in Modern Jewish Social History. 1973.

04480   GLOGOWSKI, L.
[*An Episode at the Auschwitz Concentration Camp*]. Przeglad Lekarski
(1970) 26(1):202–203.

04490   GLOGOWSKI, L.
*From "Guinea Pig" in Auschwitz to the Post of Head of the Hospital in
Birkenau.* In Auschwitz, In Hell They Preserved Human Dignity,
Anthology, Vol. 2, Part 1. Warsaw: International Auschwitz
Committee, 1971, 150–183.

04500   GLOWACKI, C.
Zmiany Pathologiczne Narzadu Rodnego U Kobiet Bylych
Wiezniarek Obozow Koncentrcyjnych. [*Gynecological Pathological
Changes in Female Concentration Camp Ex-Prisoners*]. Ginekol Pol
(1973) 44:901–906.

04510   GLOWACKI, C.
Die Biologischen Auswirkungen Von Spätfolgen Einer In Frühen
Jugend Durchagemachten Hungerdystrophie Bei Frauen, Die Im
Konzentrationslager Auschwitz-Birkenau Festgehalten Wurden. II
Ausbleiben Der Menstruation Nach Der Lagerhaft. [*The Biological
Aspects of Late Sequelae of a Hunger Dystrophy Undergone in Early
Childhood, in Women That Were Imprisoned in C.C. Auschwitz-
Birkenau. Omission of Menstruation after Camp Internment*]. VI
Internationaler Medizinischer Kongress Der F.I.R., Prague, 1976.

04520 GLOWACKI, C.
Brak Miesiaczki U Kobiet Bylych Wiezniow Obozow
Koncentracyjnych [*Amenorrhea in Female Concentration Camp
Ex-Prisoners*]. Ginekologia Pol (1976) 47:1403–1408.

04540 GLOWACKI, C.
[*Pathologic Precocious Senility in Women, Former Inmates of
Concentration Camps during World War II*]. Ginekol Pol (1973)
44(3):315–318.

04550 GOGOLOWSKA, S.
[*Health Services at the Janowska Camp*]. Przeglad Lekarski (1975)
32(1):89–96.

04560 GOLDBURG, J.B.
*The Transmittal of the Trauma of the Holocaust to Survivor Children
and American Jewish Children.* Ed.D. diss., Drake University, 1983.
Page 953 in Vol. 44/03-B of Dissertation Abstracts International.
Order No: AAD83-16265.

04570 GOLDSCHMIDT, E.P.
Over de Joodsche oorlogspleegkinderen. [*Concerning Jewish War
Orphans in Foster Families*]. Maandblad Geestelijke Volksgezondheid
1 (1946) 12:310–311.

04580 GOLDSTEIN, J.; LUKOFF, K.F.; STRAUSS, H.
A Case History of a Concentration Camp Survivor. Am O.S.E. Rev
(1951) 8:11–28.

04590 GOODMAN, J.S.
*The Transmission of Parental Trauma: Second Generation Effects of
Nazi Concentration Camp Survival.* Ph.D. diss., California School of
Professional Psychology, Fresno, 1979. Page 4031 in Vol 39/08-B of
Dissertation Abstracts International. Order No: AAD79-01805.

04600 GOTTSCHICK, J.
Psychiatrie der Kriegsgefangenschaft. [*Psychiatry of Prisoners of War*].
Stuttgart: Gustav Fischer Verlag, 1963.

04610 GOUDSMIT, W.
Leven na een oorlog . . . of: over oorlogsslachtoffers. [*Life After a
War . . . or: About War Victims*]. Maandblad Geestelijke
Volksgezondheid 27 (1972) (9):412–216.

04620 GOUKASSIAN, H.
Hungerdystrophie. [*Hunger Dystrophy*]. In Michel, M. (ed.),
Gusundheitsschäden Durch Verfolgung Und Gefangenschaft Und Ihre
Spätfolgen. Frankfurt Am Main: Röderberg Verlag, 1955, 127–134.
Also In Fichez, L.F. (ed.), Andere Spätfolgen. Austria: Verlag Der
F.I.R., 1959, Band 2, 33–40.

04630 GRAAF, De T.
*Pathological Patterns of Identification in Families of Survivors of the
Holocaust.* Isr Ann Psychiat and Rel Disc (1975) 13(4):335–363.

04640   GRAUER, H.
Psychodynamics of the Survivor Syndrome. Can Psychiat Ass J (1969)
14(6):617–622.

04650   GREENBLATT, S.
The Influence of Survival Guilt on Chronic Family Crises. J Psychol
Judaism (1978) 2(2):19–28.

04660   GREVE, W.
Die Rückgliederung Von Verfolgten: Ihre Begutachtung. [The
Rehabilitation of Persecutees: Its Evaluation]. Therapiewoche (1963)
22:1–4.

04670   GREVE, W.; RUFFIN, H.
Erfahrungen Bei Der Begutachtung Von Verfolgten. [Experiences in
the Evaluation of Persecutees]. Jahrbuch Für Psychologie Und
Psychotherapie (1963) 11:66–81.

04680   GROBIN, W.
Medical Assessment of Late Effects of National Socialist Persecution.
Can Med Ass J (1965) 92:911–917.

04690   GROEN, J.
Psychogenesis and Psychotherapy of Ulcerative Colitis. Psychosom Med
(1947) 9:151.

04700   GRØNVIK, O.; LØNNUM, A.
The Neurological Condition of Ex-Prisoners from Concentration Camps.
In Later Effects of Imprisonment and Deportation. International
Conference Organized by the World Veterans Federation. The Hague:
World Veterans Federation, 1961, 89–92.

04710   GRØNVIK, O.; LØNNUM, A.
Neurological Conditions in Former Concentration Camp Inmates. J
Neuropsychiat (1962) 4:50–54.

04720   GRØNVIK, O.; LØNNUM, A.
Neurologiske Folgetilstander Hos Tidligere Konsentrasjonsleirfanger.
[Neurological Sequelae in Concentration Camp Ex-Prisoners]. Tidsskrift
For Den Norske Lageforening (1961) 81:810–816 (808–810).
Reprinted in Tidsskr Norske Lageforening (1961) 803–816.

04730   GRUBRICH-SIMITIS, I.
[Extreme Traumatization as Cumulative Trauma; Psychoanalytic
Investigations of the Effects of Concentration Camp Experience in
Survivors and Their Children]. Psyche (1979) 33(11):991–1023. Also in
Psychoanalytic Study of the Child. New Haven: Yale University
Press, 1981, 36:415–450.

04740   GRUBRICH-SIMITIS, I.
[From Concretism to Metaphor. Thoughts on Psychoanalytic Work with
Descendants of the Holocaust Generation–On the Occasion of a New
Development]. Psyche (1984) 38(1): 1–28.

04750   GRYGIER, T.
Oppression: A Study in Social and Criminal Psychology. New York:
Grove Press, 1954.

04760   GRUNBERGER, B.
Der Antisemit und der Oedipuskomplex. [*The Anti-Semite and the Oedipus Complex*]. Psyche (1962/63) 16:255.

04770   GUTERMAN, S.S.
Alternative Theories in the Study of Slavery, the Concentration Camp, and Personality. Brit J Sociol (1975) 186:186–202.

04780   GUTT, R.W.
Remarks on the Subject of Ethics of Nazi Physicians. In Auschwitz, Inhuman Medicine, Anthology, Vol. 1, Part 2. Warsaw: International Auschwitz Committee, 1971, 205–221.

04790   GUTT, R.W.
After a Quarter of a Century. Przeglad Lekarski (1975) 32(1):212–213.

04800   GYOMROI-LUDOWYK, E.
The Analysis of a Young Concentration Camp Victim. 1. The Psychoanalytic Study of the Child (1963) 18:484–510. 2. In Zwingman, (ed.), Uprooting and After. Berlin: Springer, 1973, 291–311.

04810   HAANS, T.
Een maatschappelijke benadering van het KZ-syndroom. [*A Social Approach to the Concentration Camp Syndrome*]. In Boutellier, H. and L. Wouda (ed.), Progressieve ontwikkelingen in de psychologie (Progressive Developments in Psychology) (1981) 93–100. Published by SUA, Amsterdam. (ISBN 90–6222–071–1)

04820   HAANS, T.
Oorlogsoverlevende of psychiatriese patient, de maatschappelijke achtergronden van het KZ-syndroom. [*Survivor of the War or Psychiatric Patient, the Social Backgrounds of the CC Syndrome*]. J of Psychologie en Maatschappij (1983) 2:223–241.

04830   HAANS, T.
Oorlogsoverlevenden: teruggekeerden of slachtoffers? [*Survivors of the War: Returned People or Victims?*] In Dane, J. (ed.), Keerzijde van de Bevrijding. [*The Other side of Liberation*]. Deventer, 1984, 36–55.

04840   HACKENBROCH, M.
Die Beurteilung Degenerativer Erkrankungen Des Stützsystems Bei Ehemaligen Kriegsgefangenen Und Verfolgten. [*The Evaluation of Degenerative Diseases of the Support-System in Former Prisoners of War and in Persecutees*]. In Herberg, H.J. (ed.), Spätschäden Nach Extremebelastungen. II Internationalen Medizinisch-Juristischen Konferenz in Düsseldorf, 1969. Herford, Nicolaische Verlagsbuchhandlung, 1971, 127–133.

04850   HADJU, G.
About the Hungarian Aspects of the Medical Expert's Assessment Concerning Decrease of Working Ability in Persons Submitted to "Pseudoscientific Medical Experiments" in the Nazi Concentration Camps. Acta Med Leg Soc (Liège) (1967) 20(2):297–302.

04860 HÄFNER, H.
Psychosocial Changes Following Racial and Political Persecution. In
Soc Psychiat (1969) 47:101–117. Also in German. Bäyer, W.; Häfner,
H.; Kisker, K. P. Psychiatrie Der Verfolgten. Berlin: Springer-Verlag,
1964.

04870 HÄFNER, H.
Psychological Disturbances Following Prolonged Persecution. Soc
Psychiat (1968) 3(3):79–88.

04880 HÄFNER, H.
Psychosocial Changes Following Racial and Political Persecution. Res
Publ Ass Res Nerv Ment Dis (1969) 47:101.

04890 HAINE, J. C.
Evaluation des Séquelles Invalidantes Tardives de la Captivité Trente
Ans après le Conflict de 1940–1945. [*Evaluation of Late Disabling
Sequelae of Captivity 30 Years after the War of 1940–1945*]. Bruxelles
Med (1974) 54:639–653.

04900 HALGAS, K.
[*From the Concentration Camp in Gross-Rosen (A Physician's
Memoirs)*]. Przeglad Lekarski (1967) 23(1):197–203.

04910 HALGAS, K.
[*Trachoma at the Gross-Rosen Concentration Camp in 1943*]. Przeglad
Lekarski (1975) 32(1):167–71.

04920 HALGAS, K.
Zagadien Sanitarnych Komanda Dyhernfurth II. [*Sanitary Conditions
at the Dyhernfurth Command*]. Przeglad Lekarski (1977) 34:122–130.

04930 HALGAS, K.
[*Section For Soviet Prisoners-of-War in Auschwitz-Birkenau
Concentration Camp*]. Przeglad Lekarski (1980) 37(1):162–171.

04940 HAMMERMAN, S. I.
*Historical Awareness and Identity Development in Young Adult
Offspring of Holocaust Survivors.* Ed.D. diss., Boston University
School of Education, 1980. Page 1941 in Vol 41/05-B of Dissertation
Abstracts International.

04950 HAMMET, P. J.
Identity under Threat of Marginality. Fourth World Congress of
Psychiatry. Madrid, Spain, 1966. Proceedings.

04960 HANKE, E.
[*Memoirs of Wincenty Spaltenstein, Prisoner of the Concentration Camp
in Dachau*]. Przeglad Lekarski (1968) 24(1):110–115.

04970 HANOVER, L. A.
*Parent-Child Relationships in Children of Survivors of the Nazi
Holocaust.* Ph.D. diss., United States International University, 1981.
Page 770 in Vol. 42/02-B of Dissertation Abstracts International.
Order No: AAD81–14741.

04980 HAU, T.F.
Vergleichende Untersuchungen An Psychosomatisch Erkrankten
Jugendlichen Der Geburtsjahrgange Der Volkrieg-, Kriegsund
Nachkriegszeit. [*Comparison Studies on Psychosomatically Ill
Youngsters Born before, during and after the War*]. Prax Kinderpsychol
Kinderpsychiat 21 (1972) 6:193–200.

04990 HEFTLER, N.
Etude sur l'Etat Actuel, Psycho-Sociologique, des Enfants Nés après
le Retour de Déportation de Leurs Parents (Père, Mère, ou les Deux.
[*Investigation of the Present State of Children, Born after the
Deportation and Liberation of their Parents (Father, Mother or Both)*].
VI Congrès Médical International de la F.I.R., Prague, 1976. Also in
German in Medizinisch Untersuchungen F.I.R., 1979, 21–26.

05000 HEGER, W.
Om Norske Konsentrasjonsleir-Fangers Stilling Idag. Ettervirkninger
Og Sosiale Problemer. [*The Situation of the Norwegian Concentration
Camp Ex-Prisoners Today. Late Sequels and Social Problems*]. Hoston:
Norske Kvinners Masjonalrads Sosialskole, 1969.

05010 HEIJMANS, D.
Discutabel CBS-onderzoek naar sterfte ex-concentrationaires. [*A
Debatable CBS-Research on Mortality Rates of former Concentration
Camp Inmates*]. Nieuw Israelitisch Weekblad, 11 June 1976.

05020 HEIMREICH, W.B.
How Jewish Students View the Holocaust: A Preliminary Appraisal. In
Steinitz, L. (ed.), Living after the Holocaust: Reflections of the
Post-War Generation in America. New York: Bloch, 1975, 101–114.

05030 HELLER, D.
*Themes of Culture and Ancestry among Children of Concentration Camp
Survivors.* Psychiatry (1982) 45:247–261.

05040 HELLER, J.
Betrachtungen Über Die Wichtigsten Herz Und Gefässerkrankungen
Bei Ehemaligen Deportierten Und Interierten. Die Aussichten Ihrer
Behandlung. [*Remarks about the Most Important Cardiovascular
Diseases in Former Deportees and Internees. The Chances of Their
Treatment*]. In Fichez, L. (ed.), Andere Spätfolgen. Austria: Verlag Der
F.I.R., 1959, Band 2, 99–129.

05050 HELLER, P.
[*Evacuation from the Auschwitz Branch Camp Jaworzno*]. Przeglad
Lekarski (1980) 37(1):176–82.

05060 HELWEG-LARSEN, P.; HOFFMEYER, H.; KIELER, J.; THAYSEN,
E.H.; THYGESEN, P.; WULFF, M.H.
Sultsygdommen Og Dens Folgetilstande Hos
Koncentrationslejrfanger. [*The Starvation Disease and Its Sequelae in
Concentration Camp Prisoners*]. Ugeskrift For Lager (1949) 111:1–65.

05070   HELWEG-LARSEN, P.; HOFFMEYER, H.; KIELER, J.; THAYSEN,
J.H.; THYGESEN, P.; WULFF, M.H.
*Famine Disease in German Concentration Camps. Complications and
Sequelae.* In Acta Psychiat Neurol Scand. Copenhagen: Ejnar
Munksgaard (1952), Sup. 83. En Francais, La Maladie de Famine,
1954.

05080   HELWEG-LARSEN, P.; HOFFMEYER, H.; KIELER, J.; THAYSEN,
J.H.; WULFF, M.H.
Herz Und Gefäss-Symptome Der Hungerdystrophie. [*Cardiovascular
Symptoms of the Hunger Dystrophy*]. In Michel, M. (ed.),
Gesundheitsschäden Durch Verfolgung Und Gefangenschaft Und Ihre
Spätfolgen. Frankfurt Am Main: Röderberg Verlag, 1955, 181– 190.

05090   HELWEG-LARSEN, P.; HOFFMEYER, H.; KIELER, J.; THAYSEN,
J.H.; WULFF, M.H.
Die Hungerkrankheit In Den Deutschen Konzentrationslagern. [*The
Hunger Disease in German Concentration Camps*]. In Michel, M. (ed.),
Gesundheitsschäden Durch Verfolgung Und Gefangenschaft Und Ihre
Spätfolgen. Frankfurt Am Main: Röderberg Verlag, 1955, 256– 267.

05100   HELWEG-LARSEN, P.
Tuberkulose-Spätfolgen. [*Tuberculosis-Late Sequelae*]. In Michel, M.
(ed.), Gesundheitsschäden Durch Verfolgung Und Gefangenschaft
Und Ihre Spätfolgen. Frankfurt Am Main: Röderberg Verlag, 1955,
101– 106.

05110   HEMMENDINGER, J.
*Readjustment of Young Concentration Camp Survivors Through a
Surrogate Family Experience.* Interaction (1980) 3(3):127– 134.

05120   HEMMENDINGER, J.
A la Sortie des Camps de la Mort: Reinsertion dans la Vie. [*Coming
Out of the Camps: Return to Life*]. Isr J Psychiat Rel Sci (1981)
18(4):331– 334. Special review of author's doctoral dissertation.

05130   HENDRIKS, G.
Conclusive Remarks and Recommendations. In Israel-Netherlands
Symposium on the Impact of Persecution, Jerusalem, 1977. The
Netherlands: Rijswijk, 1979, 7– 9.

05140   HENDRIKS, G.
Het Kz-syndroom en de sociale omgeving, een korte vergelijkende
analyse over de psychische nawerkingen van de Tweede
Wereldoorlog bij vervolgden in Polen en Nederland. [*The
Concentration Camp Syndrome and the Social Surroundings, A Brief
Comparative Analysis on the Psychic Sequelae of World War II in
Persecuted People in Poland and Holland*]. Maatschappelijk Welzijn 27
(1975) 3:62– 68.

05150   HENSELER, H.
Zum Gegenwaertigen Stand Der Beurteilung Erlebnisdedingter
Spätschäden Nach Verfolgung. [*The Present State of the Evaluation of
Compensation Experiences after Persecution*]. Nervenarzt (1965)
36:333– 338.

05160   HERBERG, H.J.
The Cardiovascular Sequelae of Detention. In Later Effects of
Imprisonment and Deportaton. International Conference Organized
by the World Veterans Federation. The Hague: World Veterans
Federation, 1961, 53–56.

05170   HERBERG, H.J.
Psychische Belastungen Und Erlebnisreaktive Störungen In Der
Pathogenes Innherer Krankheiten. [*Psychic Stress and Experiential
Disturbances in the Pathogenesis of Internal Diseases*]. In Paul, H. and
H.J. Herberg (eds.), Psychische Spätschäden Nach Politischer
Verfolgung. Basel: S. Karger, 1963, 357–380.

05180   HERBERG, H.J.
Der Gegenwärtige Stand Der Beurteilung Von Gesundheitsschäden
Nach Gefangenschaft Und Verfolgung In Der Bundesrepublik
Deutschland. [*The Present State of the Evaluation of Health Damage
after Imprisonment and Persecution in the German Federal Republic*].
In Herberg, H.J. (ed.), Die Beurteilung Von Gesundheitsschäden
Nach Gefangenschaft Und Verfolgung. Internationalen
Medizinisch-Juristischen Symposiums in Köln, 1967. Herford:
Nicolaische Verlagsbuchhandlung, 1967, 12–20.

05190   HERBERG, H.J.
Die Beurteilung Von Gesundheitsschäden Nach Gefangenschaft Und
Verfolgung. Internationalen Medizinisch-Juristischen Symposiums in
Köln, 1967. [*The Evaluation of Health Damage after Internment and
Persecution*]. Herford: Nicolaische Verlagsbuchhandlung, 1967. With
papers by: Herberg, Ellenbogen, Lingens, Noodhoek-Hegt, Oyen,
Linne, Venzlaff, Weber, Hoffman, Jacob, Brost, Paul,
Paul-Mengelberg, Fischer, Dietze.

05200   HERBERG, H.J.
Die Ärztliche Beurteilung Verfolgter Im Entschädigungserfahren.
[*The Medical Evaluation of Persecuted People in the Work of
Indemnification*]. In Paul, H. and H.J. Herberg (eds.), Psychische
Spätschäden Nach Politischer Verfolgung. Basel: S. Karger, 1967,
239–252.

05210   HERBERG, H.J.
Spätschäden Nach Extremebelastungen. [*Late Damage after Extreme
Stress*]. II Internationalen Medizinisch-Juristischen Konferenz, II
Düsseldorf, 1969. Herford: Nicolaische Verlagsbuchhandlung, 1971.
With papers by: Saller, Paul, Jacob, Schenk, Venzlaff, Klimkova,
Amelunxen, Hoffman, Blaha, Lingens, Hackenbroch, Lønnum,
Eitinger, Sheps, Paul-Mengelberg, V. Baeyer, Matussek, Klange,
Dickhaut, Burgman, Lempp, Tyndel, Wangh, Hoff, Brym-Oyen, Ott.

05220   HERMAN, S.
The Meaning of Death: Experience with Survivors in Holland. Group
Analysis, Special Issue: The Survivor Syndrome Workshop,
November 1980, 33–42.

05230   HERMAN, K.; THYGESEN, P.
KZ-Syndromet Hungerdystrofiends Folgetilstand 8 ar Efter. [*The

KZ-Syndrome. The Sequelae of Hungerdystrophy Eight Years Later].
Ugeskrift For Lager. Copenhagen (1954) 116:825–836.

05240   HERMANN, K.; THYGESEN, P.
In La Déportation dans les Camps de Concentration Allemands et Ses
Sequelles. [Deportation in German Concentration Camps and its
Consequences]. F.I.R., Paris, 1954.

05250   HERMANN, K.
Die Psychischen Symptomen Des KZ Syndroms Versuch Einer
Pathogenetischen Schätzung. [*The Psychic Symptoms of the
Concentration Camp Syndrome. An Attempt at a Psychopathogenic
Evaluation*]. In Michel, M. (ed.), Gesundheitsschäden Durch
Verfolgung Und Gefangenschaft Und Ihre Spätfolgen. Frankfurt Am
Main: Röderberg Verlag, 1955, 41–47.

05260   HERS, J.F.P.
Orgaanaandoeningen bij personen deel uitmakend van het voormalig
Nederlands Verzet, de Krijgsmacht en Koopvaardij, alsmede bij
Vervolgden en Gedeporteerden tijdens de Tweede Wereldoorlog, een
follow-up studie over een periode van 33 jaar. [*The Effects on the
Organs of Former Members of the Dutch Resistance, the Army and
Merchant Service, As Well As The Persecuted and Deported During
World War II: A Follow-Up Study Over a Period of 33 Years*]. In Dane,
J., Keerzijde van de Bevrijding, Deventer, 1984, 146–174.

05270   HERTZ, D.G.; FREYBERGER, H.
*Factors Influencing the Evaluation of Psychological and Psychosomatic
Reactions in Survivors of the Nazi Persecution.* J Psychosom Res (1982)
26:83–89.

05280   HERZOG, J.M.
*The Aging Survivor of the Holocaust. Father Hurt and Father Hunger:
The Effect of a Survivor Father's Waning Years on His Son.* J Geri
Psychiat (1981) 14(2):211–223.

05290   HERZOG, J.M.
World beyond Metaphor: Thoughts on the Transmission of Trauma. In
Bergmann, M.S. and M.E. Jucovy (eds.), Generations of the
Holocaust. New York: Basic Books, 1982, 103–119.

05300   HES, J.P.
*Some Remarks on the Case of Specificity in the Administration of
Psychiatric Help.* In Ayalon, O. (ed.), The Holocaust and Its
Perseverance. Assen, 1983, 49–51.

05310   HESS-THAYSEN, E.; HESS-THAYSEN, J.
Les Problèmes Médicaux chez les Anciens Deportés. [*The Medical
Problems of Elderly Deportees*]. Copenhagen: Congresverslag, 1954.

05320   HESS-THAYSEN, E.; HESS-THAYSEN, J.
Medizinische Probleme Bei Fruheren in Deutschen
Konzentrationslager Deportierten. [*Medical Problems in Former
Deportees to German Concentration Camps*]. In Michel, M. (ed.),

Gesundheitsschäden Durch Verfolgung und Gefangenschaft Und Ihre Spätfolgen. Frankfurt: Röderberger-Verlag, 1955, 172–189.

05330 HILBERG, R.
The Nature of the Process. The Perpetrators. The Victims. In Dimsdale, J.E. (ed.), Survivors, Victims, and Perpetrators. Washington: Hemisphere Publishing, 1980, 5–54.

05340 HIRSCHFELD, M.J.
Care of the Aging Holocaust Survivor. Am J Nurs (1977) 77(7):1187–1189.

05350 HIRSCHLER, P.
Over Oorlogneuroses. [*Concerning War Neuroses*]. Ned Mil Geneesk T (1951) 6:159.

05360 HOCKING, F.
Human Reactions to Extreme Environmental Stress. Med J Austral (1965) 52:477–482.

05370 HOCKING, F.
Psychiatric Effects of Extreme Environmental Stress. Dis Nerv Syst (1970) 31(8):324–326.

05380 HOCKING, F.
Psychiatric Aspects of Extreme Environmental Stress. Dis Nerv Syst (1970) 544–545.

05390 HOCHHEIMER, W.
Vorurteilsminderung In Der Erziehung Und Die Prophylaxe Des Antisemitismus. [*Decreasing Prejudice Through Education and the Prevention of Antisemitism*]. Psyche (1962/63) 16:285.

05400 HOCHMAN, J.
On the Analysis of a Child of Holocaust Survivors with Some Notes on Countertransference Problems. Bull Southern California Psychoanal Institute and Society (1978) 33.

05410 HOEFER, C.H.
[*Concentration Camp Confinement in the Light of a Phenomenology of Alienation*]. Klin Psychol Psychopathol Psychother (1983) 31(4):333–351.

05420 HOFF, H.
Die Klinik Psychischer Verfolgungschäden. [*The Hospital of Psychic Persecution*]. In Herberg, H.J. (ed.), Spätschäden Nach Extremebelastungen. II Internationalen Medizinisch-Juristischen Konferenz in Düsseldorf, 1969. Herford: Nicolaische Verlagsbuchhandlung, 1971, 285–289.

05430 HOFFMAN, T.
Verfolgungsschäden Haftungsgrenze Und Stellenwert Psychischer Schäden Unter Beruecksichtigung Der Sonderrelungen Und Beweiserleichterungen Im Beg. [*The Importance, Limits and Evaluation of Psychological Damages as Practiced According to the Newer German Restitution Law's (Beg) Special Regulations*]. In

Herberg, H. J. (ed.), Die Beurteilung Von Gesundheitsschäden Nach Gefangenschaft Und Verfolgung. Internatinalen Medizinisch-Juristischen Symposiums in Köln, 1967. Herford: Nicolaische Verlagsbuchhandlung 1967, 58–65.

05440   HOFFMEYER, H.
Soziale Und Therapeutische Aspekte Der Spätfolgen. [*Social and Therapeutic Aspects of Late Sequelae*]. In Michel, M. (ed.), Gesundheitsschäden Und Ihre Spätfolgen. Frankfurt Am Main: Röderberg Verlag, 1955, 251–255.

05445   HOGMAN, F.
Displaced Jewish Children During World War II: How They Coped. J. Humanistic Psychology. (1983) 20(3)51–66.

05450   HOGMAN, F.
Role of Memories in World War II Orphans. Presented at the APA Symposium on Child Survivors of the Holocaust—Forty Years Later. Los Angeles, 1984. Manuscript. In J Amer Acad Child Psychiat, July 1985.

05460   HOOGENVEEN, B. N. V.
De sociale problematiek van de tweede generatie, onrecht, onschuld en onvrede. [*The Social Problems of the Second Generation, Injustice, Innocence and Discontent*]. In Psycho-sociale problematiek van de tweede generatie (2) [*Psychosocial Problems of the Second Generation*], een bundeling van de drie inleidingen gehouden op de studiedag over de psycho-sociale problematiek van de tweede generatie georganiseerd door de Stichting ICODO op 9 juni 1983. Utrecht, 1983, 20–30.

05470   HOPPE, K. D.
Persecution, Depression and Aggression. Bull Menninger Clinic (1962) 26:195–203.

05480   HOPPE, K. D.
Über Den Einfluss Der Übergangsobjekte Und Phänomene Auf Die Behandlungssituation. [*Concerning the Influence of Transitional Objects and Phenomena in Symptom Formation.*]. In G. Scheunert (ed.), Jahrbuch Der Psychoanalyse, Vol. 4. Bern, Stuttgart: Hans Huber, 1964.

05490   HOPPE, K. D.
[*Psychotherapy of Concentration Camp Victims*]. Psyche 1965 19(5):290–319.

05500   HOPPE, K. D.
Persecution and Conscience. Psychoanal Rev (1965) 52:106–116.

05510   HOPPE, K. D.
Psychotherapie Bei Konzentrationslageropfern. [*Psychotherapy with Concentration Camp Victims*]. Psyche (1965) 19:290.

05520   HOPPE, K. D.
The Psychodynamics of Concentration Camp Victims. Psychoanalytic

Forum (1966) 1:1, 76–85. Discussants: Niederland, Chodoff, Friedman, Jacobson.

05530 HOPPE, K. D.
Zum Gegenwärtigen Stand Der Beurteilung Erlebnisbedingter Spätschäden Nach Verfolgung. [*On the Present Status of Compensation and Evaluation Experiences Following Persecution*]. Nervenarzt (1966) 37:124.

05540 HOPPE, K. D.
The Emotional Reactions of Psychiatrists When Confronting Survivors of Persecution. Psychoanalytic Forum (1968)3:186–211.

05550 HOPPE, K. D.
Über Den Einfluss Der Übergangsobjekte Und Phänomene Auf Die Behandlungssituation. [*Concerning the Influence of Transitional Objects and Phenomena in Treatment*]. In Scheunert, G. (ed.), Jahrbuch Der Psychoanalyse, Vol. 4. Bern, Stuttgart: Hans Huber, 1967.

05560 HOPPE, K. D.
Psychotherapy with Concentration Camp Survivors. In Krystal, H. (ed.), Massive Psychic Trauma. New York: International Universities Press, 1968, 204–219.

05570 HOPPE, K. D.
Psychosomatic Reactions and Disorders in Survivors of Severe Persecution. Psyche (1968) 22(6):464–477.

05580 HOPPE, K. D.
Re-Somatization of Affects in Survivors of Persecution. Int J Psycho-Anal (1968) 49(2–3):324–326.

05590 HOPPE, K. D.
Symposium on Psychological Problems after Severe Mental Stress. Discussion in Lopez Ibor, J. (ed.), Proceedings, Fourth World Congress of Psychiatry, Madrid, 1966, Vol. 2. New York: Excerpta Medica Foundation, 1968.

05600 HOPPE, K. D.
Psychosomatic Reactions and Disorders in Victims of Persecution. In Lopez Ibor, J. (ed.), Proceedings, Fourth World Congress of Psychiatry, Madrid, 1966, Vol. 4, New York: Excerpta Medica Foundation, 1968.

05610 HOPPE, K. D.
Psychosomatische Reaktionen Und Erkrankungen Bei Überlebenden Schwerer Verfolgung. [*Psychosomatic Reactions and Disorders in Survivors of Severe Persecution*]. Psyche (1968) 22:464.

05630 HOPPE, K. D.
The Aftermath of Nazi Persecution Reflected in Recent Psychiatric Literature. Int Psychiat Clinics (1971) 8:169–204.

05640   HOPPE, K.D.
Chronic Reactive Aggression in Survivors of Severe Persecution. Compr
Psychiat (1971) 12(3):230–237.

05660   HOPPE, K.D.
Differing Views of Survivorship: Severed Ties. In Luel, S.A. and
P. Marcus (eds.), Psychoanalytic Reflections on the Holocaust:
Selected Essays. New York: Ktav Publishing House, 1984, 95–112.

05670   HORMUTH, S.E.; STEPHAN, W.G.
Effects of Viewing "Holocaust" on Germans and Americans: A
Just-World Analysis. J Appl Soc Psychol (1981) 11(3) 240–251.

05680   HOTTINGER, A.; GSELL, O.; UEHLINGER, E.; SALZMAN, C.;
LABHART, A.
Hungerkrankheit—Hungerodem—Hungertuberkulose. [Hunger
Disease, Hunger Edema, Hunger Tuberculosis]. Basel: Benno Schwabe,
1948.

05690   HOUTEN, Van Den, A.
Geslagen mensen, de zorg voor oorlogsgetroffenen. [Battered People,
the Assistance for War Victims]. Den Haag: Omniboek (no date)

05700   HÜBSCHMANN, H.
Tuberkulose Und Wiedergutmachung. [Tuberculosis and
Indemnification]. Beiträge Zur Klinik Der Tuberkulose (1959)
120:305–314.

05710   HÜBSCHMANN, H.
Terror Und Krankheit. [Terror and Disease]. Adv Psychosom Med
(1963) 3:28–34.

05720   HÜBSCHMANN, H.
Psychosomatik Der Erkrankungen Politisch Verfolgter.
[Psychosomatic of the Morbidity of Politically Persecuted People].
Verhandlung Der Deutschen Gesellschaft Für Innere Medizin 73.
Kongress, 1967, 696–701.

05730   HÜBSCHMANN, H.
Politische Verfolgung Als Ursache Der "Alterskrankheiten"
Bluthochdruck Und Arteriosklerose. [Political Persecution as the Cause
of Geriatric Diseases: High Blood Pressure and Arteriosclerosis]. In
Ermüdung Und Vorzeitiges Altern. Folge Von Extremebelastungen. V
Internationaler Medizinischer Kongress Der F.I.R., Paris, 1970.
Leipzig: Johann Ambrosius, 1973, 167–172.

05740   HÜBSCHMANN, H.
Die Bedeutung Der Latenz Für Die Beurteilung Von
Verfolgungsbedingten Gesundheitsschäden. [The Meaning of the
Latency for the Evaluation of Health Damage Caused by Persecution].
VI Internationaler Medizinischer Kongress Der F.I.R., Prague, 1976.

05750   HUGENHOLTZ, P.
Psychologische opmerkingen over den na-oorlogschen mens.
[Psychological Observations on the Post-War Person]. Ned T Psychol
(1947) 1:20.

05760 HUGENHOLTZ, P.
De factoren bij de instandhouding van de psychosociale problematiek van oorlogsgetroffenen. [*The Factors in Maintaining the Psychosocial Problems of War Victims*]. In Dane, J. Keerzijde van de Bevrijding. Deventer, 1984, 18–27.

05770 HUK, B.
Reihenuntersuchung Ehemaliger KZ-Ler [*Social Examinations of Concentration Camp Ex-Prisoners*]. In Michel, M. (ed.), Gesundheitsschäden Durch Verfolgung Und Gefangenschaft Und Ihre Spätfolgen. Frankfurt Am Main: Röderberg Verlag, 1955, 82–83.

05780 HUNT, R.
Entering the Future Looking Backwards (Holocaust and the Nazi Experience). Hastings Center Report (1978) 8(3)3: 5–6.

05790 HUSTINX, A.
Het existentieel emotioneel stresssyndroom. [*The Existential Emotional Stress Syndrome*]. Maandblad Geestelijke Volksgezondheid 28 (1973) 5:197–206.

05800 INBONA, J.M.
Contribution to the Study of Cardiovascular Symptoms among Former Deportees Liberated from German Concentration Camps. In Later Effects of Imprisonment and Deportation. International Conference Organized by the World Veterans Federation. The Hague: World Veterans Federation, 1961, 57–60.

05810 INBONA, J.M.
Contribution à l'Etude des Symptomes Cardiovasculaires chez les Anciens Deportés Libérés des Camps de Concentration Allemands. [*Contributions to the Study of the Cardiovascular Symptoms in Former Deportees Who Were Liberated from German Concentration Camps*]. Semaines Méd Prof (1963) 839:87–89.

05820 ILLESCU, C.C.
Die Herz Und Gefässstörungen Unter Den Bedingungen Des Hätflingslebens Und Der Unterernährung. [*Cardio-Vascular Disturbances in Conditions of Imprisonment and Malnutrition*]. In Ätio-Pathogenese Und Therapie Der Ershöpfung Und Vorzeitigen Vergreisung. IV Internationaler Medizinischer Kongress Der F.I.R. Bucharest: Verlag Der F.I.R., 1964, 269–301.

05830 IRONSIDE, W.
Conservation-Withdrawal and Action-Engagement: On a Theory of Survivor Behavior. Psychosom Med (1980) 42(1):163–175.

05840 IWASZKO, T.; KLODZINSKI, S.
[*Rebellion of Inmates Condemned to Death at Barracks 11 of the Auschwitz Concentration Camp on 28th Oct. 1942 under the Leadership of Capt. Dr. Henryk Suchnicki*]. Przeglad Lekarski (1977) 34(1):118–22.

05850 IVY, A.
Nazi Medical Crimes of a Medical Nature. J Am Med Ass (1949) 139:131–138.

05860   JABLONSKI, C.
[Mortality in the Brzeziny Ghetto]. Przeglad Lekarski (1980)
37(1):40–43.

05870   JACKMAN, N. R.
Survival in the Concentration Camp. Hum Org (1958) 17:23–26.

05880   JACOB, W.
Gesellschaftliche Voraussetzungen Zur Überwindung Der
KZ-Schäden. [Social Preconditions for Overcoming Concentration
Camp Damage]. Nervenarzt (1961) 32:542–545.

05890   JACOB, W.
Zur Beurteilung Der Zusammenhangfrage Körperllicher Und
Seelischer Verfolgungsschäden In Der Gutachtichen Praxis Des
Entschädigungsverfahrens. [Evaluation of the Question of Connection
Between Somatic and Psychic Damages Due to Persecution in the
Indemnification]. In Herberg, H.J. (ed.), Die Zur Beurteilung Von
Gesundheitsschäden Nach Gefangenschaft Und Verfolgung.
Internationalen Medizinisch-Juristischen Symposiums in Köln (1967).
Herford: Nicolaische Verlagsbuchhandlung 1967, 66–72.

05900   JACOB, W.
Erb-Unwelteinfluesse Bei "Anlageleiden" [Heredity and Environmental
Influences in "Endogenous" Diseases]. In Herberg, H.J. (ed.),
Spätschäden Nach Extremebelastungen II Internationalen
Medizinisch-Juristischen Konferenz in Düsseldorf, 1969. Herford:
Nicholaische Verlagsbuchhandlung, 1971, 29–35.

05910   JACOBS-STAM, C.M.
Oorlog, een breuk in het bestaan, achtergrond en problemen van
door de oorlog getroffenen. [War, a Rupture in the Existence
Background and Problems of Victims of the War]. Van Loghum
Slaterus: Deventer, Holland, 1981.

05920   JACOBSEN, E.
Luftencephalogrammet Ved KZ Syndromet. [The
Pneumoencephalogram in the Concentration Camp Syndrome].
Ugeskrift For Laeger (1955) 117:809–812.

05930   JAFFE, R.
Hahistaglut Hanafshit Shel Nitsolei Hamishtar Hanatzi Aharei
'Aliyatam Leyisrael. [Emotional Adaptation of Nazi Regime Survivors
after Their Immigration to Israel]. Dapim Refuiim (1962) 21:127–130.

05940   JAFFE, R.
Group Activity as a Defence Method in Concentration Camps. Isr Ann
Psychiat Rel Disc (1963) 1(2):235–243.

05950   JAFFE, R.
Dissociative Phenomena in Former Concentration Camp Inmates. Int J
Psycho-Anal (1968) 49(2–3):310–312.

05960   JAGIELSKI, S.
[Mental Development of "Muslims" (Peculiar Facies of Concentration

Camp Inmates in Their Terminal Phase)]. Przeglad Lekarski (1968) 24(1):106–9.

05970 JAGIELSKI, S.
[*Prof. Stanislaw Konopka: Three Chapters from My Life*]. Arch Hist Med (Warsz) (1983) 46(4):475–480.

05980 JAGODA, Z.; KLODZINSKI, S.; MASLOWSKI, J.
[*Laughter in a Concentration Camp*]. Przeglad Lekarski (1973) 30(1):84–99.

05990 JAGODA, Z.; KLODZINSKI, S.; MASLOWSKI, J.
[*Cultural Life at the Auschwitz Concentration Camp*]. Przeglad Lekarski (1974) 31(1):19–39.

06000 JAGODA, Z.; KLODZINSKI, S.; MASLOWSKI, J.
[*Drug Addiction at the Auschwitz Camp*]. Przeglad Lekarski (1975) 32(1):40–67.

06010 JAGODA, Z.; KLODZINSKI, S.; MASLOWSKI, J.
Stereotype Verhaltensweise Der Ehemaligen Häftlinge Des KZ Auschwitz-Birkenau. [*Behavioral Stereotypes in Former Inmates of Nazi Concentration Camps*]. Przeglad Lekarski (1976) 33(1):46–71.

06020 JAGODA, Z.
La Survie au Camp de Concentration dans l'appréciation d'anciens Prisonniers D'Auschwitz-Birkenau. [*Survival in Concentration Camp as Viewed by Former Prisoners of Auschwitz-Birkenau*]. VI Congrès Médical International de la F.I.R., Prague, 1976.

06030 JAGODA, Z.; KLODZINSKI, S.; MASLOWSKI, J.
Stereotype Verhaltensweisen Der Ehemaligen Häftlinge Des KZ Auschwitz Birkenau. [*Stereotypical Behaviour of Former Prisoners of the Concentration Camp Auschwitz-Birkenau*]. VI Internationaler Medizinischer Kongress Der F.I.R., Prague, 1976.

06040 JAGODA, Z.; KLODZINSKI, S.; MASLOWSKI, J.
Sny Wiezniow Obozu Oswiecimskiego. [*Dreams of Prisoners From Concentration Camp Auschwitz*]. Przeglad Lekarski (1977) 34:28–66.

06050 JAGODA, Z.; MASLOWSKI, J.; KLODZINSKI, S.
Przetrwanie Obozu W Olenie Bylych Wiezniow Oswiecimia-Brzezinki. [*The Survival in the Camp Evaluated by Ex-Prisoners From Auschwitz-Birkenau*]. Przeglad Lekarski (1977) 34:77–108.

06060 JAGODA, Z.; KLODZINSKI, S.; MASLOWSKI, J.
[*Friendships Struck Up at the Auschwitz Concentration Camps*]. Przeglad Lekarski (1978) 35(1):32–77.

06070 JAGODA, Z.; KLODZINSKI, S.; MASLOWSKI, J.
[*The Auschwitz Vocabulary*]. Przeglad Lekarski (1978) 35(1):78–94.

06080 JAGODA, Z.; KLODZINSKI, S.; MASLOWSKI, J.
[*Aggression and Aggressiveness in Auschwitz*]. Przeglad Lekarski (1980) 37(1):43–75.

06090   JAGODA, Z.; KLODZINSKI, S.; MASLOWSKI, J.
[Attitude of Survivors of the Auschwitz-Birkenau Camps to Their
Former Persecutors]. Przeglad Lekarski (1981) 38(1):37–62.

06100   JAGODA, Z.; KLODZINSKI, S.; MASLOWSKI, J.; WESOLOWKSA,
D.
[The Auschwitz Dictionary (C-C). A Model]. Przeglad Lekarski (1984)
41(1):62–67.

06110   JAKUBIK, A.
Pseudomedizinische Experimente In Den Hitlerschen
Konzentrationslagern. [Pseudo Medical Experiments in the Hitlerian
Concentration Camps]. Mitteilungen Der F.I.R. (1974) 3:9–14. Also in
Polish in Przeglad Lekarski (1973).

06120   JAKUBIK, A.; RYN, Z.
[Pseudomedical Experiments in Nazi Concentration Camps]. Przeglad
Lekarski (1973) 30(1):64–72.

06130   JAKUBIK, A.; RYN, Z.
[Pseudomedical Experiments in Nazi Concentration Camps. Polish
Bibliography 1945–1971]. Przeglad Lekarski (1973) 30(1):72–75.

06140   JAKUBIK, A.
[Self Image and Confinement in Hitlerite Concentration Camps.
Theoretical and Methodological Problems]. Przeglad Lekarski (1981)
38(1)15–26.

06150   JANOTA, O.
Conséquences de la Deuxième Guerre Mondiale en Tchécoslovaquie
au Point de Vue Psychiatrique. [Consequences of the Second World
War in Czechoslovakia, from a Psychiatric Point of View]. Presse
Médicale (1946) 49:667–668.

06160   JASPERS, K.
The Criminal State and German Responsibility: A Dialogue with R.
Augstein. Commentary (1966) 2:33.

06170   JEDRZEJCZAK, W.
Przewlekle Nastepstwa Psychiczne Pobytu W Hitlerowskich Obozach
Koncentracyjnych na Podstawie Badan 214 Bylych Wiezniow.
[Chronic Psychological Sequels after Incarceration in Hitlerian
Concentration Camps, Based on the Investigation of 214 Ex-Prisoners].
Ann Acad Med Stetinensis (1973) 19:537–563.

06180   JEKIELEK, W.
[Supporting Action of the "Peasant Brigade" for the Prisoners of the
Auschwitz-Birkenau Concentration Camp]. Przeglad Lekarski (1966)
22(1):120–131.

06190   JEZIERSKA, M.E.
[Problems of Small Concentration Camps]. Przeglad Lekarski (1967)
23(1):127–128.

06200   JEZIERSKA, M.E.
It Is Not Permitted to Be Sick. In Auschwitz, In Hell They Preserved

Human Dignity, Anthology, Vol. 2, Part 2. Warsaw: International Auschwitz Committee, 1971, 193–216.

06210 JEZIERSKA, M.E.
[*Sanitary Conditions Prevailing during the Evacuation of 1944–1945. (Theory and Facts)*]. Przeglad Lekarski (1978) 35(1):147–154.

06220 JEZIERSKA, M.E.
[*The Hospital in the Buchenwald Concentration Camp (According to the Archives Records for the Period of April 3, 1945 to July 20, 1945)*]. Przeglad Lekarski (1980) 37(1):76–85.

06230 JOFEN, J.
Long-Range Effects of Medical Experiments in Concentration Camps (The Effect of Administration of Estrogens to the Mother on the Intelligence of the Offspring). In Proceedings of the Fifth World Congress of Jewish Studies, The Hebrew University Mount Scopus—Givat Ram, Jerusalem, 3–11 August 1969, Vol. 2, 55–71. World Union of Jewish Studies.

06240 JORES, A.
In Dauernder Angst—Elf Jahre In Einzelhaft. [*In Continued Fear–Eleven Years in Solitary Confinement*]. In H. March (ed.), Verfolgung und Angst. Stuttgart: Ernst Klett Verlag, 1960.

06250 JUCOVY, M.E.
The Effects of the Holocaust on the Second Generation: Psychoanalytic Studies. Am J Soc Psychiat (1983) 3(1):15–20.

06260 KACYZYNSKI, A.
Gosciec U Wieznow Obozow Koncentracyjnych W Obrazie Owczesnym I Aktualnum. [*Rheumatism in Prisoners of Concentration Camps Based on Past and Present Data*]. Przeglad Lekarski (1969) 25(1):28–30.

06270 KACZYNSKI, A.
Der Gelenkrheumatismus Bei Ehemaligen Häftlingen Hitlerscher Konzentrationslager. [*Rheumatic Arthritis in Former Prisoners of Hitler-Concentration Camps*]. Mitteilungen Der F.I.R. (1975) 8:22–24.

06280 KAHANA, R.J.
The Aging Survivor of the Holocaust. Discussion: Reconciliation between the Generations: A Last Chance. J Geri Psychiat (1981) 14(2):225–239.

06290 KAHN, M.L.
Les Problèmes de la Seconde Generation. [*The Problems of the Second Generation*]. Vie Congrès Médical International de la F.I.R. Prague, 1976. Also in German, Medizinisch Intersuchungen.... Vienna: F.I.R.(1979) 27–28.

06300 KALMA, J.J.
Redt de Joden! Wat gebeurt er met de Joodse pleegkinderen? [*Save The Jews! What Happens with the Jewish Foster Children?*] Amsterdam: De Arbeiderspers, 1946.

06310   KALMA, J. J.
Wat gebeurt er met de Joodse pleegkinderen? Nogmaals: redt de
Joden! [*What Happens With the Jewish Foster Children? Once More:
Save The Jews!*]. October 1946.

06320   KAMIENSKI, B.
[*Reminiscing about the Sonderaktion Krakau*]. Przeglad Lekarski
(1976) 33(1):171–179.

06330   KAMPEN-BRONKHORST, Van, D.
De oorlog duurt voort, over de problematiek van oorlogsgetroffenen.
[*The War Goes On, On the Problems of War Victims*]. Den Haag: VUGA
1979.

06340   KANTER, I.
Extermination Camp Syndrome: The Delayed Type of Double-Bind. Int J
Soc Psychiat. 4 (1970) 16:275–282.

06350   KANTER, I.
Social Psychiatry and the Holocaust. J Psychol Judaism (1976)
1:55–66.

06370   KAROLINI, T.
Poczatki Rewiru W Gusen. [*The Beginning of the Sick Bay in the
Camp of Gusen*]. Przeglad Lekarski (1976) 33:179–183.

06390   KARR, S. D.
Second Generation Effects of the Nazi Holocaust. Ph.D. diss.,
California School of Professional Psychology, San Francisco, 1973.
Page 2935 in Vol. 35/06-B of Dissertation Abstracts International.
Order No: AAD73-30244.

06400   KASAHARA, Y.
[*Concentration Camp Syndrome*]. Nippon Rinsho (1977) 35 (Suppl
1):698–699.

06410   KATZ, C.
Tuberkulose Und Deportation. [*Tuberculosis and Deportation*]. In
Aetio-Pathogenese Und Therapie Der Erschöpfung Und Vorzeitigen
Vergreisung. IV Internationaler Medizinischer Kongress Der F.I.R.
Bucharest: Verlag Der F.I.R., 1964, 334–336.

06420   KATZ, C.
Les Problèmes de la Pathologie de la Résistance En France. [*Problems
of the Pathology of the Resistance in France*]. VI Congrès Médical
International de la F.I.R., Prague, 1976.

06430   KATZ, C.; KELEMAN, F. A.
The Children of the Holocaust Survivors: Issues of Separation. J Jewish
Communal Serv (1981) 257–263.

06440   KAV-VENAKI, S.; NADLER, S.
*Sharing the Holocaust Experience: Comparison between Two Groups of
Survivors and Their Descendants.* Presented at a Conference on the
"Second Generation": Children of Holocaust Survivors, N.Y.C., 1979.
Manuscript.

06450   KAV-VENAKI, S.; NADLER, A.
        Transgenerational Effects of Massive Psychic Traumatization: Psychological Characteristics of Children of Holocaust Survivors in Israel. Paper presented at the Fourth Annual Scientific Meeting of the International Society of Political Psychology, Mannheim, June 24–27, 1981. Manuscript.

06460   KAV-VENAKI, S.; NADLER, A.; GERSHONI, H.
        Sharing Past Traumas: A Comparison of Communication Behaviors in Two Groups of Holocaust Survivors. Int J Soc Psychiat (1983) 29(1):49–59.

06470   KEILSON, H.
        Zur Psychologie Der Jüdischen Kriegswaisen. [*On the Psychology of Jewish Orphans*]. Psychohygiene (1949)1–6.

06480   KEILSON, H.
        Vooroordeel en haat, een psychologische bijdrage tot het probleem van het anti-semitisme. [*Prejudice and Hate, A Psychological Contribution to the Problem of Anti-Semitism*]. Maandblad Geestelijke Volksgezondheid 16 (1961) 3:83–98.

06490   KEILSON, H.
        Sequentielle Traumatisierung Bei Kindern. [*Sequential Traumatization in Children*]. Forum der Psychiatrie. Stuttgart: Ferdinand Enke Verlag, 1979.

06500   KEILSON, H.
        Sequential Traumatization of Children. Dan Med Bull (1980) 27:235–237.

06510   KEILSON, H.
        Afscheid, herinnering en rouw. [*Parting, Recollection and Mourning*]. Stichting ICODO. Utrecht, Holland. In Scheiding en rouw, 16–22, 1983.

06520   KEMPINSKI, A.
        TZW. "KZ Syndrom." Proba Syntezy. [*The So-Called Concentration Camp Syndrome—An Experiment of a Synthesis*]. Przeglad Lekarski (1970) 27:18–23.

06530   KEMPINSKI, A.
        Z Niemieckich Badan Nad Nastepstwami Przebywania W Obozach Hitlerowskich. [*The German Investigations on the Sequelae of Incarceration in the Hitlerian Camps*]. Przeglad Lekarski (1972) 29:243–246.

06540   KEMPINSKI, A.
        Le Syndrome Concentrationnaire. Essai d'une Synthèse. [*The Concentration Camp Syndrome. An Attempt at Synthesis*]. Cah d'inf F.I.R. (1973) 1:3–12.

06550   KEMPINSKI, A.; KLODZINSKI, S.
        Über Die Positiven Psychischen Reaktionen Der Häftlinge. [*On the Positive Psychic Reactions of Inmates*]. Mitteilungen Der F.I.R. (1976) 10:1–7.

06560   KEMPISTY, C.
Stan Zdrowia Bylych Wieznio Ze Srodowiska Wroclawskiego. [*State of Health of Former Concentration Camp Inmates from the Wroclaw Area*]. Przeglad Lekarski (1967) 24:96–98.

06570   KEMPISTY, C.
Wyniki Badan Lekarskich Bylych Wiezniow Obozu Dla Dzieci W Lodzi. [*The Results of Sociomedical Investigations of Children of Ex-Prisoners in Lodz*]. Przeglad Lekarski (1970) 27:24–27.

06580   KEMPISTY, C.
Wyniki Socjo-Medycznych Badan Potomstwa Bylych Wiezniow Obozow Hitlerowskich. [*The Results of Sociomedical Investigations of Children of Ex-Prisoners of the Hitlerian Camps*]. Przeglad Lekarski (1973) 30:12–20.

06590   KEMPISTY, C.
Leszczynska. Z Badan Nad Plodnoscia Bylych Wiezniarek Obozow Hitlerowskich. [*Investigations of the Fertility of Female Ex-Prisoners of Hitlerian Camps*]. Przeglad Lekarski (1974) 31:58–65.

06600   KEMPISTY, C.
Ergebnisse Der 2 Sozialmedizinischer Untersuchung Der Kinder Von Eltern, Die In Hitler-Konzentrationslagern Interniert Waren. [*Experiences of the Second Social-Medical Examination of Children Whose Parents Were Prisoners in Hitler's Concentration Camp*]. Mitteilungen Der F.I.R. (1975) 8:25–26.

06610   KEMPISTY, C.
Ergebnisse Der Sozialmedizischen Untersuchung Von Personen, Die Als Kinder In Nazikonzentrationslagern Waren. [*Results of Social Medical Examinations of Persons Who Were in Nazi Concentration Camps as Children*]. Mitteilungen Der F.I.R. (1975) 8:27–29.

06620   KEMPISTY, C.; LESZCZYNSKA, Z.
Results of *Socio-Medical Studies of Persons Deported to the Third Reich as Slave Laborers*. Przeglad Lekarski (1975) 32(1):70–8.

06630   KEMPISTY, C.
Ergebnisse Der Soziomedizinischen Untersuchungen Der Nachkommenschaft Der Ehemaligen KZ-Häftlinge. [*Results of Sociomedical Examinations of Offspring of Concentration Camp Survivors*]. VI Internationaler Medizinischer Kongress Der F.I.R., Prague, 1976.

06640   KEMPISTY, C.; KRUSZCZYNSKI, K.; PILICHOWSKI, C.; SZWARC, H.
Biologische Und Oekonomische Folgen Der Deportation Und Gefangenhaltung Der Polen In Den Nazi-Konzentrationslagern. [*Biological and Economical Sequelae of Deportation and Imprisonment of Poles in the Nazi Concentration Camps*]. VI Internationaler Medizinischer Kongress Der F.I.R., Prague, 1976.

06650   KEMPISTY, C.; PIOTROWSKA, E.
Problemy Gerontologii Spolecnej W Procesie Zmian Aktywnosci

Bylych Wieznioiw Przechodzacych Na emeryture. [*Gerontological Problems during the Change of Activity in Ex-Prisoners Who Are about to Retire*]. Przeglad Lekarski (1977) 34:17–25.

06660 KEMPISTY, C.
[*Offspring of the Former Inmates of Nazi Concentration Camps*]. Przeglad Lekarski (1979) 36(1):18–25.

06670 KEMPISTY, C.
Pathogenese Der Kriegsinvalidität Und Letalität Der Ehemaligen KZ-Häftlinge. [*Causes of War, Disability and Mortality in Former Inmates of Concentration Camps*]. In Cah d'inf méd soc jurid (1983) 19:122–123.

06680 KEPINSKI, A.
Anus Mundi. In: Auschwitz, Inhuman Medicine, Anthology, Vol. 1, Part 2. Warsaw: International Auschwitz Committee, 1971, 1–12.

06690 KEPINSKI, A.
Auschwitz Reflections: The Railway Loading Platform, The Psychopathology of Decision. In Auschwitz, Anthology, Vol 3, Part 2. Warsaw: International Auschwitz Committee, 1972, 81–129.

06700 KEPINSKI, A.
[*German Studies of Sequelae of Imprisonment in Nazi Concentration Camps*]. Przeglad Lekarski (1972) 29(1):243–246.

06710 KEPINSKI, A.
A Nightmare. In Auschwitz, It Did Not End in Forty-Five, Anthology, Vol. 3, Part 2. Warsaw: International Auschwitz Committee, 1972, 241–260.

06720 KEPINSKI, A.; KLODZINSKI, S.
[*Positive Mental Activity of Inmates at Concentration Camps*]. Przeglad Lekarski (1973) 30(1):81–4.

06730 KESTENBERG, J.S.
Psychoanalytic Contributions to the Problem of Children of Survivors from Nazi Persecution. Isr Ann Psychiat Rel Disc (1972) 10:311–325.

06740 KESTENBERG, J.S.
Introductory Remarks. In Anthony, E.J. and C. Koupernik (eds.), The Child in His Family: The Impact of Disease and Death. New York: Wiley, 1973, 359–361.

06750 KESTENBERG, J.S.
Kinder Von Überlebenden Der Naziverfolgungen Psychoanalytische Beiträge. [*Children of Survivors of Nazi Persecutees. Psychoanalytic Contribution*]. Psyche (1974) 28:249–265.

06760 KESTENBERG, J.S.
[*Psychoanalysis of Children of Survivors From the Holocaust: Case Presentations and Assessment*]. J Am Psychoanal Ass (1980) 28(4):775–804.

06770   KESTENBERG, J. S.; KESTENBERG, M.
Psychoanalyses of Children of Survivors from the Nazi Persecution: The Continuing Struggle of Survivor Parents. Victimology (1980) 5(2–4):368–373.

06780   KESTENBERG, J. S.
The Psychological Consequences of Punitive Institutions. Isr J Psychiat Rel Sci (1981) 18:15–30.

06790   KESTENBERG, J. S.
The Experience of Survivor Parents. In Bergmann, M. S. and M. E. Jucovy, (eds.), Generations of the Holocaust. New York: Basic Books, 1982, 46–61.

06800   KESTENBERG, J. S.
Survivor Parents and Their Children. In Bergmann, M. S. and M. E. Jucovy (eds.), Generations of the Holocaust. New York: Basic Books, 1982, 83–101.

06810   KESTENBERG, J. S.
A Metapsychological Assessment Based on an Analysis of a Survivor's Child. In Bergmann, M. S. and M. E. Jucovy (eds.), Generations of the Holocaust. New York: Basic Books, 1982, 137–158.

06820   KESTENBERG, J. S.
Die Kinder Der Verfolgten, Ein Vergleich Zwischen Den Analysen Der Erwachsenen Und Der Kinder. [*The Children of the Persecuted, A Comparison between the Analyses of the Adults and the Children*]. Arbeitshafte Kinder Psychoanal (1982) 2, 33–59.

06830   KESTENBERG, J. S.
History's Role in the Psychoanalyses of Survivors and Their Children. Am J Soc Psychiat (1983) 3(1):24–28.

06840   KESTENBERG, J. S.; GAMPEL, Y.
Growing Up in the Holocaust Culture. Isr J Psychiat Rel Sci (1983) 20(1–2):129–146.

06850   KESTENBERG, J. S.
Discussion. Presented at the APA Symposium on Child Survivors of the Holocaust—40 Years Later. Los Angeles 1984. Manuscript.

06860   KESTENBERG, M.
Discriminatory Aspects of the German Indemnification Policy: A Continuation of Persecution. In Bergmann, M. S. and M. E. Jucovy (eds.), Generations of the Holocaust. New York: Basic Books, 1982, 62–77.

06870   KESTENBERG, M.
Die Diskriminierende Praxis In Der Wiedergutmachung. [*The Discriminating Practice in the Reparations*]. Arbeitshafte Kinderpsychoanal (1982) 2:183–214.

06880   KESTENBERG, M.
Legal Aspects of Child Persecution. Presented at the APA Symposium

on Child Survivors of the Holocaust—Forty Years Later. Los Angeles 1984. Manuscript. In J Amer Acad Child Psychiat July 1985.

06890   KIEDRZYNSKA, W.
[*A Logbook of Deliveries at the Ravensbruck Camp*]. Przeglad Lekarski (1976) 33(1):95-104.

06900   KIELER, J.; THYGESEN, P.
Endrocrine Glands. In Helweg-Larsen, P. et al., Famine Disease in German Concentration Camps. Complications and Sequels. Acta Psychiat Neurol Scand. Sup. 83. Copenhagen: Ejnar Munksgaard, 1952, 199–206.

06910   KIELER, J.; THAYSEN, J.H.
Behandlung Der Hungerkrankheit. [*Treatment of Hunger Disease*]. In Michel, M. (ed.), Gesunheitsschäden Durch Verfolgung Und Gefangenschaft Und Ihre Spätfolgen. Frankfurt Am Main: Röderberg Verlag, 1955, 324–331.

06920   KIELER, J.
Immediate Reactions to Capture and Deportation. Dan Med Bull (1980) 27(5):217–220.

06930   KIELKOWSKI, R.
The Plaszow Concentration and Compulsory Labour Camp. Przeglad Lekarski (1971) 27(1):23–26.

06940   KIETA, M.
The S.S. and Police Institute of Hygiene in Auschwitz. Przeglad Lekarski (1980) 37(1):144–146.

06950   KIJAK, M.; FUNTOWICZ, S.
The Syndrome of the Survivor of Extreme Situations: Definitions, Difficulties, Hypotheses. International Rev Psychoanal (1982) 9(1) 25–33.

06960   KINSLER, F.
Second Generation Effects of the Holocaust: The Effectiveness of Group Therapy in the Resolution of the Transmission of Parental Trauma. J Psychol Judaism (1981) 6:53–67.

06970   KINSTON, W.; ROSSER, R.
Disaster: Effects on Mental and Physical State. J Psychosom Res (1974) 18(6):437–456.

06980   KISKER, K.P.
Die Psychiatrische Begutachtung Der Opfer Nazionalsozichistischer Verfolgung. [*Compensation of Nazi Persecution*]. Koyr, d. Psychiatria et Neurologia. Dresden: Geselloch, 1961.

06990   KLEBANOW, D.
Hunger Und Psychische Erregung Als Ovar-Und Keimschädigung. [*Hunger and Psychic Arousal as the Cause of Ovarial and Gonadal Disturbances*]. Geburtshilfe Und Frauenheilkunde (1948) 8:812–820.

07000   KLEIN, F.
[*Janusz Korczak–Physician and Educator–A Symbol of Humanity in Action for Today's Medical and Pedagogical Practice*]. Off Gesundheitswes (1984) 46(5):244–248.

07010   KLEIN, H.J.; ZELLERMAYER, J.; SHANAN, J.
Former Concentration Camp Inmates on a Psychiatric Ward. Arch Gen Psychiat (1963) 8:334–342.

07020   KLEIN, H.
Problems in the Psychotherapeutic Treatment of Israeli Survivors of the Holocaust. In Krystal, H. (ed.), Massive Psychic Trauma. New York: International Universities Press, 1968, 233–248.

07030   KLEIN, H.
Children and Social Catastrophe. American Psychoanalytic Association Annual Meeting, Boston 1968.

07040   KLEIN, H.
Families of Survivors in the Kibbutz: Psychological Studies. In Krystal, H. and W. Niederland (eds.): Psychic Traumatization, Vol. 8. Boston: Little, Brown, 1971.

07050   KLEIN, H.
Holocaust Survivors in Kibbutzim: Readaptation and Reintegration. Isr Ann Psychiat Rel Disc (1972) 10:(1):78–91.

07060   KLEIN, H.
Children of the Holocaust: Mourning and Bereavement. In Anthony, E.J. and C. Koupernik (eds.), The Child in His Family: The Impact of Disease and Death. New York: Wiley, 1973, 393–409.

07070   KLEIN, H.; REINHARZ, S.
Adaptation in the Kibbutz of Holocaust Survivors and Their Families. In Miller, L. (ed.), Mental Health in Rapid Social Change. Jerusalem: Academic Press, 1972.

07080   KLEIN, H.
Child Victims of the Holocaust. J Clin Child Psychol (1974) Summer:44–47.

07090   KLEIN, H.
Delayed Affects and After-Effects of Severe Traumatization. Isr Ann Psychiat Rel Disc (1974) 12(4):293–303.

07100   KLEIN, H.; LAST, U.
Cognitive and Emotional Aspects of the Attitudes of American and Israeli Youth towards the Victims of the Holocaust. Isr Ann Psychiat Rel Disc (1974) 12(2):111–131.

07110   KLEIN, H.; LAST, U.
Attitudes toward Persecutor Representations in Children of Traumatized and Nontraumatized Parents: Cross-Cultural Comparison. In Adolescent Psychiatry: Developmental and Clinical Studies (eds. S.C. Feinstein and P.L. Giovacchini) Chicago: U. of Chicago Press, 1978. Adoles Psychiat (1978) 6:224–238.

07120 KLEIN, H.
Some Theoretical and Clinical Aspects of the Impact of the Holocaust on Survivors and Their Families. In Israel-Netherlands Symposium on the Impact of Persecution, Jerusalem, 1977. The Netherlands: Rijswijk, 1979, 38–44.

07130 KLEIN, H.
The Meaning of the Holocaust. Isr J Psychiat Rel Sci (1983) 20(1–2):119–128.

07140 KLEIN, O.
Vliv Kocentracniho Tabora na Ethicky Charackter Zidovske Mladeze. [*Effect of a Concentration Camp on the Ethical Character of Young Jewish People*]. Thesis, Prague, 1948.

07150 KLEINPLATZ, M. M.
The Effects of Cultural and Individual Supports on Personality Variables among Children of Holocaust Survivors in Israel and North America. Ph.D. diss., University of Windsor, 1980. Page 1114 in Vol. 41/03-B of Dissertation Abstracts International.

07160 KLEPINSKI, A.
[*The So-Called Concentration Camp Syndrome. An Attempt at Synthesis*]. Przeglad Lekarski (1970) 26(1):18–23.

07170 KLIMKOVA-DEUTSCHOVA, E.
Chronicka Progresivni Astenie Jako Soucast Vlivu Valecnych Utrap Na Nervovou Soustavu. [*The Chronic Progressive Asthenia as Part of the War Stress on the Nervous System*]. Prakticky Laker (1961) 41:145–152.

07180 KLIMKOVA-DEUTSCHOVA, E.
Neurologische Beiträge Zur Diagnostik Und Therapie Der Folgezustaende Des Krieges. [*Neurological Contribution to the Diagnosis and Therapy of States Resulting from the War*]. In Die Behandlung Der Asthenie Und Der Vorzeitigen Vergreisung Bei Ehemaligen Widerstanskämpfern Und KZ Häftlingen. III Internationaler Medizinischer Konferenz. Luettich: Verlag Der F.I.R., 1961, 51–62.

07190 KLIMKOVA-DEUTSCHOVA, E.
Neurologische Aspekte Der Kriegsfolgen Und Ihre Dynamik. [*Neurological Aspects of War Sequels and Their Dynamics*]. In Aetio-Pathogenese Und Therapie Der Erschöpfung Und Vorzeitigen Vergreisung. IV Internationaler Medizinischer Kongress Der F.I.R. Bucharest: Verlag Der F.I.R., 1964, 541–554.

07200 KLIMKOVA-DEUTSCHOVA, E.
Neurologische Und Psychische Folgezustände Des Krieges Und Der Verfolgung Bei Kindern Und Jugendlichen. [*Neurological and Psychic States in Children and Juveniles, Resulting from the War and Persecution*]. In Herberg, H. J. (ed.), Spätschäden Nach Extremebelastungen. II Internationalen Medizinisch-Juristischen Konferenz in Düsseldorf, 1969. Herford: Nicolaische Verlagsbuchhandlung, 1971, 252–262.

07210   KLIMKOVA-DEUTSCHOVA, E.
Beitrag Zu Den Erkrankungen Des Stützsystems. [*Contributions to the Morbidity of the Support-System*]. In Herberg, H. J. (ed.), Spätschäden Nach Extremebelastungen. II Internationalen Medizinisch-Juristischen Konferenz in Düsseldorf, 1969. Herford: Nicolaische Verlagsbuchhandlung, 1971, 134–135.

07220   KLIMKOVA-DEUTSCHOVA, E.
Neurologische Aspekte Von Veränderungen Der Knochenstruktur Und Intrakranialen Kalzifikationen Nach Hunger. [*Neurological Aspects of Changes in the Structure of the Bones and Intracranial Calcification after Hunger*]. In Ermüdung Und Vorzeitiges Altern. Folge Von Extremebelastungen. V Internationaler Medizinischer Kongress Der F.I.R., Paris, 1970. Leipzig: Johann Ambrosius, 1973, 39–48.

07230   KLIMKOVA-DEUTSCHOVA, E.
Folgen Des Krieges Bei Weiteren Generationen. [*War Consequences in Later Generations*]. VI Internationaler Medizinische Kongress Der F.I.R., Prague, 1976.

07240   KLIMKOVA-DEUTSCHOVA, E.
Die Situation Der Kinder In Der Welt. [*The Situation of the Children in the World*]. Mitteilungen Der F.I.R. (1978) 14:7–10.

07250   KLIMKOVA-DEUTSCHOVA, E.
Folgen Des Krieges Bei Weiteren Generationen. [*The Sequels of WW II in Further Generations*]. Medizinische Untersuchungen Der Spätfolgen Des Krieges. VI Internationaler Medizinischer Kongress Der F.I.R., Vienna, 1979, 3–12.

07260   KLODZINSKI, S.
Untersuchungen Über Lungentuberkulose Bei Ehemaligen Häftlingen Des KZ Lagers Auschwitz. [*Examinations of Lung Tuberculosis in Former Internees of the Concentration Camp Auschwitz*]. In Aetio-Pathogenese Und Therapie Der Erschöpfung Und Vorzeitigen Vergreisung. IV Internationaler Medizinischer Kongress Der F.I.R. Bucharest: Verlag Der F.I.R., 1964, 288–290.

07270   KLODZINSKI, S.
Zbrodnicze Doswiadczenia Farmakologiczne Na Wiezniach Obozu Koncentracyjnego W Oswiecimiu. [*Criminal Pharmacological Experiments on Prisoners of the Auschwitz Concentration Camp*]. In Piaty Zeszyt Poswiecony Zagadnieniom Lekarskim Okresu Hitlerowskiej Okupacji. Przeglad Lekarski (1965), 21(1):40–46.

07280   KLODZINSKI, S.
Dur Wysypkowy W Obozie Oswiecim I. [*Typhus Exanthematicus in the Camp of Auschwitz*]. In Piaty Zeszyt Poswiecony Zagadnieniom Lekarskimk Okresu Hitlerowskiej Okupacji. Przeglad Lekarski (1965), 21(1):46–48.

07290   KLODZINSKI, S.
Cel I Metodyka Badan Lekarskich Bylych Wiezniow Hitlerowskich

Obozow Koncentracyjnych. [*Goal and Methods of Medical Examination of Ex-Prisoners From Hitlerian Concentration Camps*]. In Piaty Zeszyt Poswiecony Zagadnieniom Lekarskimk Okresu Hitlerowskiej Okupacji. Przeglad Lekarski (1965) 21(1):34–36.

07300 KLODZINSKI, S.; KUTYBA, J.
Wstepne Wywiki Badan Stanu Zdrowia 100 Bylych Wieznio Hitlerowskich Obozow Koncentracyjnych. [*Preliminary Results of a Health Investigation of 100 Ex-Prisoners of Hitlerian Camps*]. Przeglad Lekarski (1966) 23:47–48.

07310 KLODZINSKI, S.
[*Pseudo-Medical Experiments on Tuberculosis in Hitler's Concentration Camps (Activities of Kurt Heissmeyer)*]. Przeglad Lekarski (1968) 36(10):1070–1072.

07320 KLODZINSKI, S.
[*Dr. Stefan Pizlo, Prisoner No. 333 of the Auschwitz Concentration Camp*]. Przeglad Lekarski (1970) 26(1):258–260.

07330 KLODZINSKI, S.
The Contribution of the Polish Health Service to Save the Life of the Prisoners in the Auschwitz Concentration Camp. In Auschwitz, In Hell They Preserved Human Dignity, Anthology, Vol. 2, Part 2. Warsaw: International Auschwitz Committee, 1971, 58–96.

07340 KLODZINSKI, S.
Criminal Pharmacological Experiments on Inmates of the Concentration Camp in Auschwitz. In Auschwitz, Inhuman Medicine, Anthology, Vol. 1, Part 2. Warsaw: International Auschwitz Committee, 1971, 13–45.

07350 KLODZINSKI, S.
"Sterilization" and Castration with the Help of X-rays in the Auschwitz Concentration Camp. In Auschwitz, Inhuman Medicine, Anthology, Vol. 1, Part 2. Warsaw: International Auschwitz Committee, 1971, 46–79.

07360 KLODZINSKI, S.
Phenol in the Auschwitz-Birkenau Concentration Camp. In Auschwitz, Inhuman Medicine, Anthology, Vol. 1, Part 2. Warsaw: International Auschwitz Committee, 1971, 99–119.

07370 KLODZINSKI, S.
Criminal Experiments with Tuberculosis Carried Out in Nazi Concentration Camps. In Auschwitz, Inhuman Medicine, Anthology, Vol. 1, Part 2. Warsaw: International Auschwitz Committee, 1971, 163–184.

07380 KLODZINSKI, S.
SS-Men in the Auschwitz "Health Service." In Auschwitz, Inhuman Medicine, Anthology, Vol. 1, Part 2. Warsaw: International Auschwitz Committee, 1971, 185–204.

07390 KLODZINSKI, S.
The Purpose and Methodology of Medical Examinations of Former Prisoners of Nazi Concentration Camps. In Auschwitz, It Did Not End

in Forty-Five, Anthology, Vol. 3, Part 1. Warsaw: International
Auschwitz Committee, 1971, 67–75.

07400   KLODZINSKI, S.
Verbrecherische Tuberkulose-experimente Im Konzentrationslager
Neuengamme: Die Tätigkeit Von Kurt Heissmeyer. [*Criminal
Experiments with Tuberculosis in the Concentration Camp
Neuengamme: The Activity of Kurt Heissmeyer*]. In Ermüdung Und
Vorzeitiges Altern. Folge Von Extremebelastungen. V Internationaler
Medizinischer Kongress Der F.I.R., Paris, 1970. Leipzig: Johann
Ambrosius, 1973, 347–348.

07410   KLODZINSKI, S.
Cel I Metodyka Badan Lekarskich Bylych Wiezniow Hitlerowskich
Obozow Koncentracyjnych. [*Goal and Methods of Medical
Examination of Ex-Prisoners from Hitlerian Camps*]. Przeglad Lekarski
(1972) 29:15–21.

07420   KLODZINSKI, S.
Swoisty Stan Chorobowy Po Przebyciu Obozow Hitlerowskich.
[*Specific Diseases after Incarceration in Hitlerian Camps*]. Przeglad
Lekarski (1972) 29:15–21.

07430   KLODZINSKI, S.
[*Pharmacy at the Women's Concentration Camp of Birkenau*]. Przeglad
Lekarski (1976) 33(1):90–95.

07440   KLODZINSKI, S.
[*Dr. Zofia Kaczkowska*]. Przeglad Lekarski (1977) 34(1):220–222.

07450   KLODZINSKI, S.
[*Sabotage at the SS Institute of Hygiene at the Buchenwald Camp. Dr.
Marian Ciepielowski*]. Przeglad Lekarski (1977) 34(1):141–145.

07460   KLODZINSKI, S.
[*Professor Janina Kowalczykowa*]. Przeglad Lekarski (1980)
37(1):196–200.

07470   KLODZINSKI, S.
[*Dr. Czeslaw Lutynski*]. Przeglad Lekarski (1980) 37(1):200–203.

07480   KLODZINSKI, S.
[*Victims of Nazi Persecutions in the Light of Expert Judicial Opinion*].
Przeglad Lekarski (1981) 38(1):221–224.

07490   KLODZINSKI, S.
[*The Pathology of Work in Auschwitz-Birkenau*]. Przeglad Lekarski
(1984) 41(1):37–54.

07500   KLODZINSKI, S.
[*A Few Remarks about the K-Z Syndrome*]. Przeglad Lekarski (1984)
41(1):17–21.

07510   KLODZINSKI, S.
[*Zbigniew Sobieszczanski, M. D.*]. Przeglad Lekarski (1984)
41(1):131–136.

07520   KLUGE, E.
Über Die Folgen Schwere Häftzeiten. [*On the Sequelae of Severe Incarceration*]. Nervenarzt (1958) 29:462–465.

07530   KLUGE, E.
Über Den Defektcharakter Von Dauerfolgen Schwerer Häftzeiten. [*Organic Defects as Chronic Sequelae of Extreme Imprisonment*]. Medizinische Sachverständige (1961) 57:185–187.

07540   KLUGE, E.
Defektzustände Nach Schweren Häftzeiten, Insbesondere Nach KZ Haft. [*On Impairment after Severe Incarceration, Mainly in Concentration Camps.*]. In Paul, H. and H.J. Herberg (eds.), Psychische Spätschäden Nach Politischer Verfolgung. Basel: S. Karger, 1963, 85–94.

07550   KLUGE, E.
Über Ergebnisse Bei Der Begutachtung Verfolgter. [*Results of Evaluations of Persecutees*]. Nervernarzt (1965) 36:321.

07560   KLUGE, E.
Über Das Problem Der Psychotherapie Bei Chronischen Verfolgungsschäden. [*The Problem of Psychotherapy in Chronic Damage Due to Persecution*]. In Herberg, H.J. (ed.), Spätschäden Nach Extremebelastungen. II Internationalen Medizinisch-Juristischen Konferenz in Düsseldorf, 1969. Herford: Nicolaische Verlagsbuchhandlung, 1971, 187–189.

07570   KLUGE, E.
Über Dauerfolgen Schwerer Häftzeiten Unter Besonderer Berücksichtigung Hirnorganischer Störungen. [*Permanent Sequels of Severe Internment, With Special Emphasis on Organic Brain Damage*]. In Ermüdung Und Vorzeitiges Altern. Folge Von Extremebelastungen. V Internationaler Medizinischer Kongress Der F.I.R., Paris, 1970. Leipzig: Johann Ambrosius, 1973, 189–194.

07580   KLUGE, E.
Das Problem Der Chronischen Schädigung Durch Extremebelastungen In Der Heutigen Psychiatrie. [*The Problem of Chronic Damage through Massive Stress in Contemporary Psychiatry*]. Fortschritte Der Neurol Psychiat (1972) 40:1–30.

07590   KLUVERS, E.; KLUVERS, I.
Jouw oorlog—mij een zorg. [*Your War—I Don't Care*]. Baarn: In Den Toren 1979.

07600   KLUYSKENS, P.
Social Aspects of Camp Pathology. In Experts Meeting on the Later Effects of Imprisonment and Deportation. Oslo, 1960. Paris: World Veterans Federation, 1960, 131–135.

07610   KLUYSKENS, P.
Legal Aspects of Camp Pathology. In Experts Meeting on the Later Effects of Imprisonment and Deportation. Oslo, 1960. Paris: World Veterans Federation, 1960, 137–142.

07620   KLUYSKENS, P.
Legal Aspects of the Problem. Comparative Report. In Later Effects of
Imprisonment and Deportation. International Conference Organized
by the World Veterans Federation. The Hague: World Veterans
Federation, 1961, 167–177.

07630   KOENIG, W.
Chronic or Persisting Identity Diffusion. Am J Psychiat (1964)
120:1081–1084.

07640   KOENIG, W.
Über Behandlungsergebnisse Der Chronisch-Reaktiven Depression
Und Anderer Psychischer Verfolgungsschäden. [*Results of the
Treatment of Chronic Reactive Depression and Other Psychiatric
Disturbances due to Persecution*]. Excerpta Med Int Cong Ser No. 150
(1966) 1816–1818.

07650   KOEVARY, H.L.
A Search For Home: The Road to Israel. In Steinitz, L. (ed.), Living
after the Holocaust: Reflections by the Post-War Generation in
America. New York: Bloch, 1975.

07660   KOLLE, K.
Psychosen Als Schädigungsfolgen. [*Psychoses as Sequelae of Damage*].
Fortschritte Der Neurol Psychiat (1958) 26:101–120.

07670   KOLLE, K.
Die Opfer Der Nationalsozialistischen Verfolgung In Psychiatrischer
Sicht. [*The Victims of the National-Socialist Persecution in the Light of
Psychiatry*]. Nervenarzt (1958) 29:148–158.

07680   KONING, DE, P.P.J.
*What Psychotherapists Have against Working with People Who Were
Persecuted during World War 2.* Israel-Netherlands Symposium on the
Impact of Persecution. 2. Dalfsen, Amsterdam, 14–18 April 1980. The
Netherlands: Rijswijk, 1981, 49–54.

07690   KORANYI, E.K.
A Theoretical View of the Survivor Syndrome. Dis Nerv Sys (1969)
30:115–118.

07700   KORANYI, E.K.
Psychodynamic Theories of the "Survivor Syndrome." Canad Psychiat
Ass J (1969) 14(2):165–174.

07710   KORCZYNSKA, A.
[*Contribution to the Problem of Help to the Prisoners of the
Auschwitz-Birkenau Concentration Camp*]. Przeglad Lekarski (1980)
37(1):113–118.

07720   KORNHUBER, H.
Psychologie und Psychiatrie der Kriegsgefangenschaft. [*The
Psychology and Psychiatry of Prisoners of War*]. In Ruhle, H. (ed.),
Psychiatrie der Gegenwart, Vol. 3. Berlin: Springer, 1961.

07730   KOSCIUSZKOWA, J.
Children in the Auschwitz Concentration Camp. In Auschwitz, In Hell
They Preserved Human Dignity, Anthology, Vol. 2, Part 2. Warsaw:
International Auschwitz Committee, 1971, 217–224.

07740   KOWALSKI, S.
Wstepne Wyniki Badan Bylych Wiezniow Hitlerowskich Obozow
Kocentracyjnych. [*Preliminary Results of an Investigation of
Ex-Prisoners from Hitlerian Concentration Camps*]. Przeglad Lekarski
(1968) 25:54–55.

07750   KRAL, V.A.
*An Epidemic of Encephalitis in the Concentration Camp Terezin
(Theresienstadt) during the Winter 1943–1944.* J Nerv Men Dis (1947)
105:403–413.

07760   KRAL, V.A.
O Epidemii Encefalitidy V Terezinskem Ghetu. [*On the Epidemic of
Encephalitis in the Ghetto of Terezin*]. Casopisu Lekaru Ceskych (1948)
87:1–15.

07770   KRAL, V.A.
Beobachtungen Bei Einer Grossen Enzephalitisepidemie.
[*Observations on a Large Epidemic of Encephalitis*]. Schw Arch Neurol
U Psychiat (1949) 64:281–328.

07780   KRAL, V.A.
Psychiatric Observations under Severe Chronic Stress. Am J Psychiat
(1951) 108:185–192.

07790   KRAL, V.A.; PAZDER, L.H.; WIGDOR, B.T.
Long-Term Effects of a Prolonged Stress Experience. Can Psychiat Ass J
(1967) 12:175–181.

07800   KRAUS, O.; KULKA, E.
Tovarna na Smrt, Dokument o Osvetimi [*Death Factory, A Document
on Auschwitz*]. Prague, 1963.

07810   KRELL, R.
Holocaust Families: The Survivors and Their Children. Comprehensive
Psychiat (1979) 20:560–568.

07820   KRELL, R.; RABKIN, L.Y.
*The Effects of Sibling Death on the Surviving Child: A Family
Perspective.* Fam Process (1979) 18:471–477.

07830   KRELL, R.
Family Therapy with Children of Concentration Camp Survivors. Am J
Psychother (1982) 36:513–522.

07840   KRELL, R.
*Aspects of Psychologic Trauma in Holocaust Survivors and Their
Children.* In Grobman, A. and D. Landes (eds.), Genocide: Critical
Issues of the Holocaust. Chappaqua, New York: Rossell Books, 1983,
371–380.

07850   KRELL, R.
Reverberations of the Holocaust in Survivor Families. Presented at the
Congress of the International Network of Children of Jewish
Holocaust Survivors, 27 May 1984. CUNY, New York. Manuscript.

07860   KRELL, R.
*Holocaust Survivors and Their Children: Comments on Psychiatric
Consequences and Psychiatric Terminology.* Comprehensive Psychiat
(1984) 25(5):521–528.

07870   KRELL, R.
The Therapeutic Value of Documenting Child Survivors. Presented at
the APA Symposium on Child Survivors of the Holocaust Forty Years
Later–Los Angeles, 1984. J Amer Acad Child Psychiat July 1985.

07880   KRELL, R.
Introduction to "Child Survivors of the Holocaust: 40 Years Later."
Presented at the APA Symposium on Child Survivors of the
Holocaust Forty Years Later. Los Angeles, 1984. J Amer Acad Child
Psychiat July 1985.

07890   KREN, G.M.
Psychohistory and the Holocaust. J Psychohist (1979) 6:409–417.

07900   KREN, G.M.; RAPPOPORT, L.
The Holocaust and the Crisis of Human Behavior. New York, London:
Holmes & Meier, 1980.

07910   KRET, J.
The Doctors Found a Way Out. In Auschwitz, In Hell They Preserved
Human Dignity, Anthology, Vol. 2, Part 1. Warsaw: International
Auschwitz Committee, 1971, 76–106.

07920   KRETOWSKI, J.; KILLAR, M.; ZNOSKO, K.; KARBOWSKI, J.;
KOSCIK-GRENDA, M.
[*Social and Medical Aid Provided to Combatants in the Bialystock
Area*]. Przeglad Lekarski (1981) 38(1):30–33.

07930   KREUZER, W.
Über Beziehungen Zwischen Köperlichen Noxen Und Psychischen
Dauerschäden Nach Schweren Häftzeiten. *On the Relationship
between Physical Noxious Stimuli and Psychic Permanent Damage after
Severe Imprisonment*]. Diss., Mainz, 1972.

07940   KREUZER, W.
Internationale Untersuchungen Über Psychische Spätschäden
[*International Examination of Psychic Late Damage*]. Mitteilungen Der
F.I.R. (1975) 9:21–32.

07950   KREUZER, W.
Über Beziehungen Zwischen Köperlichen Noxen Und Psychischen
Dauerschäden Nach Schweren Häftzeiten. [*The Relation between
Physical and Psychic Permanent Damage after Severe Incarceration*].
Nervenarzt (1975) 46:291–296.

07960 KROPVELD, J.
Het KZ-Syndroom. [*The Concentration Camp Syndrome*]. Thesis, Universiteit van Amsterdam, 1983.

07970 KRYSTAL, H.
The Late Sequelae of Massive Psychic Trauma. Theme of the First Studies of Concentration Camp Survivors. The Second Wayne State University Workshop on the Late Sequelae of Massive Psychic Traumatization. Detroit, 1964.

07980 KRYSTAL, H.
Psychic Sequelae of Massive Psychic Trauma. Lopez Ibor, J. (ed.). Proceedings, Fourth World Congress of Psychiatry, Madrid, 1966, Vol. 2. New York: Excerpta Medica Foundation, 1968.

07990 KRYSTAL, H.
Massive Psychic Trauma. New York: International Universities Press, 1968. With chapters by: Bychowski, Danto, Hoppe, Klein, Krystal, Meerloo, Niederland, Petty, Sterba, Tanay, Venzlaff, Dorsey, Lifton, Souris.

08000 KRYSTAL, H.; CATH, S.
Children and Social Catastrophe: Sequelae in Survivors and the Children of Survivors. American Psychoanalytic Association, Fall Meeting, 19 December 1968, New York City. Manuscript.

08010 KRYSTAL, H.; PETTY, T.A.
The Psychological Complications of Convalescence. In Krystal, H. (ed.), Massive Psychic Trauma. New York: International Universities Press, 1968, 227–296.

08020 KRYSTAL, H.; PETTY, T.A.
The Dynamics of the Adjustment to Migration. Psychiat Q (Suppl 37) 1963, 118.

08030 KRYSTAL, H.
Trauma: Considerations of Its Intensity and Chronicity 2. In Krystal, H. and G. Niederland (eds.), Psychic Traumatization. Boston: Little, Brown, 1970, 11–28.

08040 KRYSTAL, H.
Review of the Findings and Implications of This Symposium. Int Psychiat Clin (1971) 8:217–229.

08050 KRYSTAL, H.; NIEDERLAND, W.G.
(Eds.). *Psychic Traumatization: After Effects in Individuals and Communities.* Int Psychiat Clin, Vol. 8. Boston: Little, Brown, 1971.

08060 KRYSTAL, H.
Trauma and Affects. Psychoanalytic Study of the Child (1978) 33:81–116.

08070 KRYSTAL, H.
The Aging Survivor of the Holocaust. Integration and Self-Healing in Post-traumatic States. J Geri Psychiat (1981) 14(2):165–189.

08080   KRYSTAL, H.
Integration and Self-Healing in Post-Traumatic States. In Luel, S.A. and P. Marcus (eds.), Psychoanalytic Reflections on the Holocaust: Selected Essays. New York: Ktav Publishing House, 1984, 113–134.

08090   KRZYWICKI, J.
Stan Uzebienie U Bylych Wiezniow Obozow Hitlerowskich. [*The Dental Status of Ex-Prisoners of Hitlerian Camps*]. In Piaty Zeszyt Poswiecony Zagadnieniom Lekarskim Okresu Hitlerowskiej Okupacji. Przeglad Lekarski (1965) 21(1):36–37.

08100   KRZYWICKI, J.
Gebissuntersuchungen Bei Personen Die Als Kinder Und Jugendliche in Haft Waren. [*Examinations of the Jaws in Persons Who as Children or Adolescents Were in Concentration Camp Imprisonment*]. Vienna, F.I.R. 1979, 83–84.

08110   KUDEJKO, J.
[*Tuberculosis Luposa Following an Experimental Vaccination at the Concentration Camp of Majdanek*]. Przeglad Dermatol (1972) 59(1):43–45.

08120   KUFFEL, E.
[*Last Days at the Ebensee Concentration Camp*]. Przeglad Lekarski (1970) 26(1):236–238.

08130   KUHN, E.V.; BRODAN, V.; HONZAK, R.; RYSANEK, K.; VOJTECHNOSKY, M.
Metabolische Auswirkung Des Schlafentzugs [*Metabolic Effect of Sleep Deprivation*]. IV Internationaler Medizinischer Kongress Der F.I.R., Prague, 1976.

08140   KULISIEWICZ, A.
[*Psychopathology of Music and Songs in Nazi Concentration Camps*]. Przeglad Lekarski (1974) 31(1):39–45.

08150   KULISIEWICZ, A.
[*Further Contributions to the Problems of Psychopathology of Music and Songs in Nazi Camps*]. Przeglad Lekarski (1975) 32(1):33–40.

08160   KULISIEWICZ, A.
[*Music and Songs as a Factor of Self-Defence Among Inmates of Nazi Concentration Camps*]. Przeglad Lekarski (1977) 34(1):66–77.

08170   KULISIEWICZ, A.
[*Music and Songs as an Instrument of Self-Defence in Nazi Concentration Camps*]. Przeglad Lekarski (1979) 36(1):38–50.

08180   KULSCAR, I.S.
The Psychopathology of Adolf Eichmann. In Lopez Ibor, J. (ed.), Proceedings, Fourth World Congress of Psychiatry, Madrid, 1966. New York: Excerpta Medica Foundation, 1968, 1687–1689.

08190   KUNDRATS, A.; GEALE, H.
Attribution of Meaning to Life in Extremis. Dissertation Abstracts International (1983) Vol. 44(1-B)290.

08200 KUPERSTEIN, E.
Adolescents of Parent Survivors of Concentration Camps: A Review of Literature. J Psychol and Judaism (1981) 6(1):7–22.

08210 KURTH, W.
Zur Frage Der Chronischen Dauerbelastung Bei Verfolgten Mit Der Folge Der Frühalterung. [*The Question of Chronic Stress in Persecutees with the Consequences of Premature Aging*]. In Ermüdung Und Vorzeitiges Altern. Folge Von Extremebelastungen. V Internationaler Medizinischer Kongress Der F.I.R., Paris, 1970. Leipzig: Johann Ambrosius, 1973, 198–200.

08220 KURTH, W.
Späte Schäden Bei In Kindheit Bzw. Jugend Verfolgter. [*Delayed Damage in Survivors Who Were Persecuted during Childhood or Youth*]. VI Internationaler Medizinischer Kongress Der F.I.R., Prague, 1976.

08230 KURTH, W.
Späte Schäden Bei in Kindheit. Jugend Verfolgter. [*Delayed Damage in Survivors Who Were Persecuted During Childhood or Youth*]. Mediz Untersuchungen Der Spätfolgen Des Krieges Und Des NS-Regimes Bei Jugendlichen Und Kindern Von Ehemaligen KZ-Häftlingen Und Verfolgten. Vienna: F.I.R., 1979, 13–20.

08240 KUZAK, Z.
Nachtwachter. [*Nightwatcher*]. Przeglad Lekarski (1979) 36(1):159–62.

08250 KUZAK, Z.
[*Spiritual Experiences of a Prisoner*]. Przeglad Lekarski (1981) 38(1):159–162.

08260 KYLE, N.; HOPPE, K.
Religiosity and Ethnocentric Idealism in Survivors of Severe Persecution. International Psychological Congress, London, 1969.

08270 LACH-KAMINI'NSKA, J.
[*In Nazi Prisons and Concentration Camps (1943–1945)*]. Przeglad Lekarski (1969) 25(1):167–72.

08280 LAMY, M.; LAMOTTE, M.; LAMOTTE-BARRILLON, S.
Osteopathies de Carence Observées chez les Déportés Libérés des Camps de Dénutrition Allemands, Hospitalisés à l'Ile de Mainau. [*Osteopathy Observed in Deportees Who Were Liberated in Extermination Camps and Treated in "Ile De Mainau"*]. Révue du Rhumatisme et des Maladies Ostéo-Articulaires.

08290 LANDAU, A.
Schlafkur Bei Chronischer Asthenie Und Vorzeitiger Vergreisung Bei Ehemaligen Deportierten Und Internierten. [*Sleeping Cure in Chronic Asthenia and Premature Senility in Ex-Deportees and Prisoners*]. In Die Behandlung Der Asthenie Und Der Vorzeitigen Vergreisung Bei Ehemaligen Widerstanskämpfern Und KZ Häftlingen. III Internationale Medizinische Konferenz. Luettich: Verlag Der F.I.R., 1961, 63–67.

08300   LANGE, A.
Re-attributie in de directieve gezinstherapie met een
oorlogsslachtoffer. [*Restructuring in Directive Family Therapy with a
War Victim*]. Tijdschr Direktieve Ther 4 (1982) 288–303.

08310   LANGE, A.
Directieve psychotherapie bij oorlogsgetroffenen. [*Directive
Psychotherapy with War Victims*]. In Dane, J., Keerzijde van de
bevrijding [*The Other Side of Liberation*]. Deventer, 1984, 118–144.

08320   LANGEVELD, M.J.
Gunstige verwerking van ongunstige ervaringen in de
levensgeschiedenis o.a. bij oorlogskinderen, enige aspekten van de
klinischpedagogische benaderingswijze in onderzoek en behandeling.
[*Positive Reworking of Unfavourable Experiences in the Lifehistory of
A.O. War Children, Some Aspects of the Clinical Pedagogical Approach
in Research and Treatment*]. (Mededelingen der Koninklijke
Nederlandse Akademie van Wetenschappen, afd. Letterkunde, nieuwe
reeks deel 39, no. 4).

08330   LANGEVELD, M.J.
Favourable Assimilation of Profound Psychic Shock. Acta
Pseudopsychiatr (1977) 43(1):7–14.

08340   LAREBEYRETTE, De J.
Der Infarkt Und Andere Gefagssstörungen In Hinkunft Vorhersehbar
Und Daher Vermeidbar. [*Cardial Infarct and Other Vascular Diseases
Can Be Predicted and Thus Prevented*]. In Die Behandlung Der
Asthenie Und Der Vorzeitigen Vergreisung Bei Ehemaligen
Widerstanskämpfern Und Häftlingen. III Internationale Medizinische
Konferenz. Luettich: Verlag Der F.I.R. (1961) 83–96.

08350   LAST, U.; KLEIN, H.
Impact de l'Holocauste: Transmission aux Enfants du Vécu des
Parents. [*Impact of the Holocaust: Transmission of Parental Experience
to the Children*]. Evolution Psychiat (1981) 46(2):373–388.

08360   LATKOWSKI, B. DE; NAJWER, P.; ZALEWSKI, P.
Etude et Estimation oto-Laryngologique des Anciens Prisonniers des
Camps de Concentration Soumis aux Experiences Pseudo-Medicales.
[*Oto-Laryngological Investigations in Ex-Concentration Camp Prisoners
Submitted to Pseudo-Medical Experiments*]. VI Congrès Medical
International de la F.I.R., Prague, 1976.

08370   LAUB, D.; AUERHAHN, N.C.
*A Generation After: Reverberations of Genocide: Its Expressions in the
Conscious and Unconscious of Post-Holocaust Generations.* In Luel,
S.A. and P. Marcus (eds.), Psychoanalytic Reflections on the
Holocaust: Selected Essays. New York: Ktav Publishing House, 1984.

08380   LAUFER, M.
The Analysis of a Child of Survivors. In Anthony, E.J. and C.
Koupernik (eds.), The Child in His Family: The Impact of Disease
and Death. New York: Wiley, 1973, 263–273.

08390 LAZNICKA, M.
Pozdni Nasledky Valky Na Zdravi Prislusniku Druheho Odboje V
Dynamickem Vyvoji 25 Let. [*The Late Sequelae of War on the Health
of Freedom Fighters. Dynamic Evolution during 25 Years*]. Casopis
Lekaru Ceskych (1973) 112:129–133.

08400 LAZNICKA, M.
Ergebnisse Einer 23 Jährigen Beobachtung Des Gesundheitszustands
Von Teilnehmern An Der Tschechoslowakischen
Widerstandsbewegung Im 2. Weltkrieg in Einem Landkreis. [*Results
of a 23 Years Health Observation of Czechoslovak Resistance Fighters in
WW II in a Rural Area*]. In Ermüdung Und Vorzeitiges Altern. Folge
Von Extremebelastungen. V Internationaler Medizinischer Kongress
Der F.I.R., Paris, 1970. Leipzig: Johann Ambrosius, 1973, 349–361.

08410 LAZNICKA, M.
Spätfolgen Des Krieges An Der Gesundheit Von Teilnehmern Am
Zweiten Tschechoslowakischen Widerstandskampf In Der
Dynamischen Enfaltung Von Dreissig Jahren. [*The Late Sequelae of
War on the Health of Participants of the Second Czechoslovak
Resistance Fight. A Dynamic Folow Up of 30 Years*]. III Internationaler
Medizinischer Kongress, Prague, 1976.

08420 LAZNICKA, M.
[*State of Health in Members of Czechoslovakia's 2nd World War
Resistance Movement as Followed Up in One District Over A Period of
33 Years (Author's Translation)*]. Cas Lek Cesk (1979)
118(49):1518–1522.

08430 LEDERER, W.
Entwurzelungsdepression Ohne Depression. Fettleibigkeit Und
Andere Psychosomatische Depressions-Äquivalente. [*Depression of
Uprooting Without Depression. Obesity and Other Psychosomatic
Equivalents of Depression*]. Nervenartz (1965)36:118–122.

08440 LEDERER, W.
Persecution and Compensation. Theoretical and Practical Implications
of the "Persecution Syndrome." Arch Gen Psychiat (1965)
12:464–474.

08450 LEGROS, J.J.; FRANCHIMONT, P.; CLAESSENS, J.J.
Profil Neuroendocrine de l'Ancien Prisonnier de Guerre (P.G.)
Hospitalisé. [*The Neuroendocrinal Profile of Hospitalized Ex-Prisoners
of War*]. VI Congrès Médical International de la F.I.R., Prague, 1976.

08460 LEHMAN, M.
[*Survivor of Inhumane Nazi Treatment Discusses Aftermath at Seminar
Here*]. NIH Record (1966) 18(16).

08470 LEHNERT, G.; SZADOWSKI, D.; VALENTIN, H.; SCHALLER, K.H.
Spätfolgen Nach Extremen Lebensverhältnissen. Untersuchungen Zu
Fragen Der Voralterung Und Einer Beeinträchtigung Des
Andrenokortikalen Regelkreises. Arbeit Und Gesundheit.
Medizinische Schriftenreihe Des Bundesministeriums Für Arbeit Und

Sozialordnung. [*Late Sequelae after Extreme Life Situations. Investigations on the Premature Senility and the Influence on the Adrenocortical System*]. Stuttgart: Georg Thieme Verlag, 1970.

08480   LEKKERKERKER, E. C.
Oorlogspleegkinderen. [*War Foster Children*]. Maandblad Geestelijke Volksgezondheid 1 (1946) 10:227–236.

08490   LEKOVA, L.
Die Verbreitung Des Diabetes Unter Den Widerstandskämpfern Des Kreises Plovdiv. [*The Distribution of Diabetes among Resistance Fighters in the County of Plovdiv*]. VI Internationaler Medizinischer Kongress Der F.I.R., Prague, 1976.

08500   LELIEFELD, H.
Immateriele hulpverlening aan oorlogsgetroffenen. [*Non-material Assistance to War Victims*]. Maandblad Geestelijke Volksgezondheid 33 (1978) 12:883–887.

08510   LELIEFELD, H.
Overlevenden van het concentratiekamp Dachau 1945–1980, een orienterend onderzoek naar ziekte, sterfte, doodsoorzaken en gebruik van wettelijke regelingen. [*Survivors of the Concentration Camp Dachau 1945–1980, An Orienting Research for Disease, Mortality, Causes of Death and the Use of Compensation Laws*]. NIPG/TNO projekt 540, deelrapport I, Leiden, 1980. Uitg Nederlands Instituut voor Praeventieve Gezondheidszorg TNO.

08520   LELIEFELD, H.
The Impact of Persecution. Review. Israel-Netherlands Symposium on the Impact of Persecution. 2, Dalfsen, Amsterdam, 14–18 April 1980. The Netherlands: Rijswijk, 1981, 15–18.

08530   LELIEFELD, H.
Nederlandse gevangenen van het concentratiekamp Dachau 1941–1979, onderzoek naar mortaliteit en doodsoorzaken. [*Dutch Prisoners of the Concentration Camp Dachau, 1941–1979, Research On Mortality and Causes of Death*]. Deelrapport 2. Leiden, 1982.

08540   LEMPP, R.
Die Bedeutung Organischer Und Psychischer Insulte In Krieg Und Verfolgung Während Der Kindheit Und Jugend. [*The Importance of Organic and Psychic Traumatization of Children and Adolescents during the War and Persecution*]. In Herberg, H. J. (ed.), Spätschäden Nach Extremebelastungen. II Internationalen Medizinisch-Juristischen Konferenz in Düsseldorf, 1969. Herford: Nicolaische Verlagsbuchhandlung, 1971, 241–251.

08550   LEMPP, R.
Extremebelastungen in Kindes—Und Jugendalter. [Über Psychosoziale Spätfolgen Nach Nationalsozialistischer Verfolgung in Kindes-und Jugendalter Anhand Von Aktengutachten]. [*Extreme Stress in Children and Youth.*] Bern/Stuttgart/Wien: Hans Huber, 1979.

08560   LEON, G.R.; BUTCHER, J.N.; KLEINMAN, M.; GOLDBERG, A.;
        ALMAGOR, M.
        *Survivors of the Holocaust and Their Children: Current Status and
        Adjustment*. J Personality and Soc Psych (1981) 41:503–516.

08570   LESNIAK, R.; ORWID, M.; SZYMUSIK, A.; TEUTSCH, A.
        Psychiatrische Studien An Ehemaligen Häftlingen Des
        Konzentrationslagers Auschwitz. [*Psychiatric Studies in
        Ex-Concentration Camp Prisoners*]. In Ätio-Pathogenese Und Therapie
        Der Erschöpfung Und Vorzeitigen Vergreisung. IV Internationaler
        Medizinischer Kongress Der F.I.R. Bucharest: Verlag Der F.I.R., 1964,
        351–357.

08580   LESNIAK, R.
        Poobozowe Zmiany Osobowosci Bylych Wiezniow Obozu
        Koncentracyjnego Oswieci-Brzezinka. [*Personality Changes after
        Imprisonment in the Concentration Camp of Auschwitz-Birkenau*]. In
        Piaty Zeszyt Poswiecony Zagadnieniom Lekarskimk Okresu
        Hitlerowskiej Okupacji. Przeglad Lekarski (1965) 21(1):13–20.

08590   LESNIAK, R.; ORWID, M.; SZYMUSIK, A.; TEUTSCH, A.;
        GATARSKI, J.; DOMINIK, M.; MITARSKI, J.;
        *Review of the Cracow Psychiatric Studies of Former Prisoners of
        Concentration Camps*. Anali Bolnice Dr. M. Stojanovic (1971)
        10:207–209.

08600   LESNIAK, R.; ORWID, M.; SZYMUSIK, A.; TEUTSCH, A.;
        GATARSKI, J.; DOMINIK, M.
        Resumee Der Krakower Psychiatrische Untersuchungen Ehemaliger
        Konzentrationslagerhäftlinge. [*Review of the Cracow Psychiatric
        Investigations of Ex-Concentration Camp Prisoners*]. In Ermüdung Und
        Vorzeitiges Altern. Folge Von Extremebelastungen. V Internationaler
        Medizinischer Kongress Der F.I.R., Paris, 1970. Leipzig: Johann
        Ambrosius, 1973, 201–203.

08610   LESNIAK, R.; MASLOWSKI, J.
        [*Psychiatric Problems in Nazi Concentration Camps in the Works of
        Antoni Kepinski*]. Przeglad Lekarski (1974) 31(1):13–18.

08620   LESNIAK, R.; LESNIAK, E.
        Ucieczki Z Obozow Koncentracyjnych. Analiza
        Psychiatryczno-Psychologiczna. [*Escapees From Concentration Camps.
        A Psychiatric-Psychological Analysis*]. Przeglad Lekarski (1976)
        33:17–24.

08630   LESNIAK, E.; LESNIAK, R.; RYN, Z.
        [*The Auschwitz Theme in the Works of Antoni Klepinski*]. Przeglad
        Lekarski (1983) 40(12):849–854.

08640   LESZCZYCKA, J.
        [*Professor Izydor Stella-Sawicki at Sachsenhausen*]. Przeglad Lekarski
        (1979) 36(1):144–146.

08650   LESZCZYCKA, S.
        Report of a Midwife from Auschwitz. In Auschwitz, In Hell They

Preserved Human Dignity, Anthology, Vol. 2, Part 2. Warsaw: International Auschwitz Committee, 1971, 181–192.

08660   LETOURMY, R.
Die Procainlangtherapie Bei Der Vorzeitigen Vergreisung Der Ehemaligen Deportierten Und Bei Seniler Asthenie. [*Procain Treatment of Premature Senility in Ex-Deportees and of Senile Asthenics*]. In Die Behandlung Der Asthenie Und Der Vorzeitigen Vergreisung Bei Ehmaligen Widerstanskämpfern Und KZ Häftlingen. III Internationale Medizinische Konferenz. Luettich: Verlag Der F.I.R., 1961, 203–220.

08670   LEVAV, I.; ABRAMSON, J.H.
Emotional Distress among Concentration Camp Survivors–A Community Study in Jerusalem. Psychol Med (1984) 14(1):215–218.

08680   LEVINE, H.B.
Toward a Psychoanalytic Understanding of Children of Survivors of the Holocaust. Psychoanalyt Q (1982) 51(1):70–92.

08690   LEVINGER, L.
Psychiatrische Untersuchungen In Israel An 800 Fällen Mit Gesundheitsschäden-Forderungen Wegen Nazi-Verfolgung. [*Psychiatric Investigations in Israel of 800 Persons Claiming Health Restitution because of Persecution by the Nazis*]. Nervenarzt (1962) 33:75–80.

08700   LICHTMAN, H.G.
Children of Survivors of the Nazi Holocaust: A Personality Study. Ph.D. diss., Yeshiva University, 1983. Page 3532 in Vol. 44/11-B of Dissertation Abstracts International. Order No: AAD84-05004.

08705   LIFTON, R.J.
Jews as Survivors in History and Human Survival, New York: Random House (1970) 195–207.

08710   LIFTON, R.J.; OLSEN, E.
The Human Meaning of Total Disaster. The Buffalo Creek Experience. Psychiat (1976) 39:1–18.

08720   LIFTON, R.J.
Witnessing Survival. Soc (1978) 40–44.

08730   LIFTON, R.J.
Survivor Experience and Traumatic Syndrome. In The Broken Connection. New York: Simon and Schuster, 1979, 163–178.

08740   LIFTON, R.J.
Victimization and Mass Violence. In The Broken Connection. New York: Simon and Schuster, 1979, 302–334.

08750   LIFTON, R.J.
The Concept of the Survivor. In Dimsdale, J.E. (ed.), Survivors, Victims and Perpetrators. Washington: Hemisphere Publishing, 1980, 106–125.

08760   LIFTON, R.J.
On the Consciousness of Holocaust. Psychohist Rev (1980) 9(1):3–22.

08770   LIFTON, R.J.
On Death and Holocaust: Some Thoughts on Survivors. Group
Analysis, Special Issue: The Survivor Syndrome Workshop.
November 1980, 13–23.

08790   LIFTON, R.J.
Medicalized Killing in Auschwitz. Psychiatry (1982) 45:283–297. Also
in Luel, S.A. and P. Marcus (eds.), Psychoanalytic Reflections on the
Holocaust. Holocaust Awareness Institute, Center for Judaic Studies,
University of Denver, and Ktav Publishing House, New York, 1984.

08800   LIFTON, R.J.
The Doctors of Auschwitz: The Biomedical Vision. Psychohist Rev
(1983) 11(2–3):36–46.

08810   LINDY, J.D.; GRACE, M.C.; GREEN, B.L.
Survivors: Outreach to a Reluctant Population. Am J Orthopsychiat
(1981) 51(3):468–478.

08820   LINGENS, E.
Expert Examinations of Psychic Damages Attributable to Political
Persecution. In Later Effects of Imprisonment and Deportation.
International Conference Organized by the World Veterans
Federation. The Hague: World Veterans Federation, 1961, 111–112.

08830   LINGENS, E.
KZ-Häftling Und Gesellschaft. [Concentration Camp Survivors and the
Society]. In Paul, H. and H.J. Herberg (eds.), Psychische Spätschäden
Nach Politischer Verfolgung. Basel: S. Karger, 1963, 21–36.

08840   LINGENS, E.
Die Situation in Österreich. [The Situation in Austria]. In Herberg,
H.J. (ed.), Die Beurteilung von Gesundheitsschäden Nach
Gefangenschaft Und Verfolgung. Internationalen
Medizinisch-Juristischen Symposiums in Köln, 1967. Herford:
Nicolaische Verlagsbuchhandlung, 1967, 21–28.

08850   LINGENS, E.
Das Problem Der "Herrschenden Lehrmeinung" Im
Begutachtungsverfahren Aus Medizinischer Sicht. [The Problem of the
"Accepted View" and Medical Experts Role]. In Herberg, H.J. (ed.),
Spätschäden Nach Extremebelastungen. II Internationalen
Medizinisch-Juristischen Konferenz in Düsseldorf, 1969. Herford:
Nicolaische Verlagsbuchhandlung, 1971, 293–297.

08860   LINGENS, E.
Die Begutachtung Arteriosklerotischer Herzkreislaufleiden.

[*Evaluation of Arteriosclerotic Vascular Diseases*]. In Herberg, H.J. (ed.), Spätschäden Nach Extremebelastungen. II Internationalen Medizinisch-Juristische Konferenz in Düsseldorf (1969). Herford: Nicholaische Verlagsbuchhandlung, 1971, 115–118.

08870 LINNE, M.
Aus Der Entschädigungspraxis Zum Begschlussgesetz. [*Some Examples of Restitution According to the German Restitution Laws*]. In Herberg, H.J. (ed.), Die Beurteilung Von Gesundheitsschäden Nach Gefangenschaft Und Verfolgung. Internationalen Medizinisch-Juristischen Symposiums in Köln, 1967. Herford Germany: Nicholaische Verlagsbuchhandlung, 1967, 46–51.

08880 LIPKOWITZ, M.H.
The Child of Two Survivors. A Report of an Unsuccessful Therapy. Isr Ann Psychiat Rel Disc (1973) 11:141–155. Also in Psyche (1974) 28:231–248.

08890 LIPZIG, F.S.
Psychotherapy with Adolescent Children of Concentration Camp Survivors. J Contemp Psychother (1972).

08900 LITYNSKI, N.
[*Dr. Szczepan Wacek—Physician, Soldier, Patriot*]. Arch Hist Med (Wars) (1980) 43(4):445–452.

08910 LOBZOWSKI, W.
[*Preliminary Results of Medical Examinations of Former Inmates of Hitler's Concentration Camps. (Province of Katowice)*]. Przeglad Lekarski (1970) 26(1):28–29.

08920 LØCHEN, E.A.
Psychometric Patterns. In Strøm, A. (ed.), Norwegian Concentration Camp Survivors. Oslo: Universitetsforlaget, New York: Humanities Press, 1968, 132–155.

08930 LØNNUM, A.
An Analytical Survey of the Literature Published on the Delayed Effects of Internment in Concentration Camps and Their Possible Relation to the Nervous System. In Experts Meeting on the Later Effects of Imprisonment and Deportation, Oslo, 1960. Paris: World Veterans Federation, 1960, 21–53.

08940 LØNNUM, A.
Om KZ Syndromet. [*On the Concentration Camp Syndrome*]. Nordisk Med (1963) 69:480–484.

08950 LØNNUM, A.
Neurological Disorders. In Strøm, A. (ed.): Norwegian Concentration Camp Survivors. Oslo: Universitetsforlaget, New York: Humanities Press, 1968, 85–123.

08960 LØNNUM, A.
Das Norwegische Kriegsopfergesetz Von 1968-Eine Follow Up Studie.

[*The Norwegian Restitution Law of 1968. A Follow Up Study*].
Manuscript.

08970   LØNNUM, A.; OYEN, O.
Über Die Neuen Kriegspensionerungsgesetz In Norwegen. [*On the New Norwegian Law of War Pensions*]. In Ermüdung Vorzeitges Altern. Folge Von Extremebelastungen. V Internationaler Medizinischer Kongress Der F.I.R., Paris, 1970. Leipzig: Johann Ambrosius, 1973, 361–365.

08980   LØNNUM, A.
Neurologische Stoerungen Bei Norwegischen Konzentrationslagerhaeftlingen. [*Neurological Disturbances in Norwegian Ex-Concentration Camp Prisoners*]. In Herberg, H.J. (ed.), Spätschäden Nach Extremebelastungen. II Internationalen Medizinisch-Juristischen Konferenz in Düsseldorf (1969). Herford: Nicholaische Verlagsbuchhandlung, 1971, 153–164.

08990   LØNNUM, A.
Wirbelsauelenspätschäden Nach Multiplen Traumen. [*Diseases in the Columna Vetebralis after Multiple Traumatizations*]. In Herberg, H.J. (ed.), Spätschäden Nach Extremebelastungen. II Internationalen Medizinisch-Juristische Konferenz in Düsseldorf, 1969. Herford: Nicholaische Verlagsbuchhandlung, 1971, 136–138.

09000   LOEWENBERG, P.
The Psychohistorical Origins of the Nazi Youth Cohort. Am Hist Rev (1971) 76:1457–1502.

09010   LOHMAN, H.M.; ROSENKOTTER, L.
Psychoanalyse In Hitlerdeutschland. Wie War Es Wirklich? [*Psychoanalysis in Hitler-Germany. Where Was It Actually?*] Psyche (1982) 36(11):961–988.

09020   LORE, S.
Jewish Holocaust Survivors' Attitudes toward Contemporary Beliefs about Themselves. Ph.D. diss., Fielding Institute, 1983. Dissertation Abstracts International. Vol. 44, no 6, p 504.

09030   LORENZER, A.
Zum Begriff Der "Traumatischen Neurose." [*The Problem of "Traumatic Neurosis"*]. Psyche (1966) 20:481–492.

09040   LORENZER, A.
Some Observations on the Latency of Symptoms in Patients Suffering from Persecution Sequelae. Int J Psycho-Anal (1968) 49:316–318.

09050   LORSKA, D.
Block Ten in Auschwitz. In Auschwitz, Inhuman Medicine, Anthology, Vol. 1, Part 2. Warsaw: International Auschwitz Committee, 1971, 80–98.

09060   LOWIN, R.G.
Cross-Generational Transmission of Pathology in Jewish Families of Holocaust Survivors. Ph.D. diss., California School of Professional

Psychology, San Diego, 1983. Page 3533 in Vol. 44/11-B of
Dissertation Abstracts International. Order No. AAD84-04702.

09070   LUCHTERHAND, E. G.
Prisoner Behavior and Social System in Nazi Concentration Camps.
Ph.D. diss., University of Wisconsin—Madison, 1953. Page 250 in Vol.
W1953.

09080   LUCHTERHAND, E. G.
*Survival in the Concentration Camp: An Individual or a Group
Phenomenon?* In Rosenberg, B.; I. Gerver and F. W. Howton, (eds.),
Mass Society in Crisis: Social Problems and Social Pathology. New
York: Macmillan, 1964.

09090   LUCHTERHAND, E. G.
The Gondola-Car Transports. Int J Soc Psychiat (1966/67) 13:1–28.

09100   LUCHTERHAND, E. G.
Identity Transformations in Survivors of Nazi Camps. A Preliminary
Report on a Longitudinal Study. Manuscript.

09110   LUCHTERHAND, E. G.
Prisoner Behavior and Social System in the Nazi Concentration Camps.
Int J Social Psychiatry (1967) 13:245–264.

09120   LUCHTERHAND, E. G.
*Early and Late Effects of Imprisonment in Nazi Concentration Camps;
Conflicting Interpretations in Survivor Research.* Soc Psychiat (1970)
5:102–110.

09130   LUCHTERHAND, E. G.
*Sociological Approaches to Massive Stress in Natural and Man-Made
Disasters.* Int Psychiat Clin (1971) 8:29–53.

09140   LUCHTERHAND, E. G.
*Social Behavior of Concentration Camp Prisoners: Continuities and
Discontinuities with Pre and Postcamp Life.* In Dimsdale, J. E. (ed.),
Survivors, Victims and Perpetrators. Washington: Hemisphere
Publishing, 1980, 259–283.

09150   LUDOWYK-GYOMROI, E.
The Analysis of a Young Concentration Camp Victim. The
Psychoanalytic Study of the Child. New York: International
Universities Press, 1963, 18:484–510.

09160   LUDZKI, M.
Children of Survivors. Jewish Spectator (1977) 2(3):41–43.

09170   LUEL, S. A.; MARCUS, P.
(Eds.). *Psychoanalytic Reflections on the Holocaust.* Holocaust
Awareness Institute, Center for Judaic Studies, University of Denver,
and New York: Ktav Publishing House, 1984.

09180   LUEL, S. A.
Living with the Holocaust: Thoughts on Revitalization. In Luel, S. A.

and P. Marcus (eds.), Psychoanalytic Reflections on the Holocaust:
Selected Essays. New York: Ktav Publishing House, 1984, 169–178.

09190 LUNGERSHAUSEN, E.; MATIAR-VAHAR, H.
Erlebnisreaktive Psychische Dauerschäden Nach
Kriegsgefangenschaft Und Deportation. [*Psychological Responses to
Compensation Following Captivity and Deportation*]. Nervenarzt (1968)
39:123.

09200 LUSTIGMAN, M. M.
*The Fifth Business: Survival as a Way of Life. An Investigation of
Concentration Camp Survivors.* Ph.D. diss., York University (Canada),
1974. Page 6976 in Vol 36/10-A of Dissertation Abstracts
International.

09210 LUTHE, R.
Erlebnisreaktiver Persönlichkeitswandel Als Begriff Der
Begutachtung Im Entschädigungsrecht. [*Personality Changes as a
Reaction to Life Events. A Problem in Expert Statements and Restitution
Law*]. Nervenarzt (1968) 39:465–467.

09220 LUTHE, R.
Die Determinationsstruktur Von Persönlichkeitsfehaltung Und Ihre
Beurteilung Im Wiedergutmachungsrecht. [*Psychopathological
Behaviour and Its Evaluation According to the Restitution Law*].
Fortschritte Der Neurol Psychiat (1970) 38:165–192.

09230 MACIEJEWSKI, Z. M.
*Results of Gynecologic Examinations of Former Women Inmates Living
in Koszalin.* Przeglad Lekarski (1975) 32(1):67–70.

09240 MAHKOTA, S.
*Health Problems of Fighters in the People's Liberation War of
Yugoslavia.* In Later Effects of Imprisonment and Deportation.
International Conference Organized by the World Veterans
Federation. The Hague: World Veterans Federation, 1961, 124–125.

09250 MAKOWSKI, A.
[*Reminiscences of a Physician from the Concentration Camps in
Monowice, Buchenwald, and Zwieberg-Langenstein*]. Przeglad Lekarski
(1967) 23(1):212–222.

09260 MAKOWSKI, A.
[*First Ward of Internal Medicine in the Hospital of the Concentration
Camp in Buna-Monowice*]. Przeglad Lekarski (1969) 25(1):71–75.

09270 MAKOWSKI, A.
Niektore Osiagniecia Oroanizacyjne Szpitala Obozowego W
Monowicach. [*Some Specific Traits in the Organization of the Sick Bay
in Monowice (Auschwitz III)*]. Przeglad Lekarski (1970) 17:165–168.

09280 MAKOWSKI, A.
[*Health Problems at the Buna-Monowice Concentration Camp in the
Light of Existing Documents*]. Przeglad Lekarski (1972) 29(1):45–51.

09290   MALLER, O.
The Late Psychopathology of Former Concentration Camp-Inmates.
Psychiat Neurol (1964) 148:140–177.

09300   MANGIAMELI, G. C.
Interpretation Cybernetique des Hallucinations chez les Survivants.
[*Cybernetical Interpretation of Survivor's Hallucinations*]. VI Congrès
Médical International de la F.I.R., Prague, 1976.

09310   MANIAKOWNA, M.
[*In the Auschwitz Concentration Camp Block No. 11*]. Przeglad
Lekarski (1970) 26(1):208–212.

09320   MANT, A. K.
Genocide. J Forensic Sci Soc (1978) 18(1–2):13–17.

09330   MARCH, H.
Zur Frage Der Neurosen Begutachtung Ein Kasuistischer Beitrag.
[*Expert Statements in Neuroses Description of a Case History*].
Medizinische Wochenschrift (1959) 10:428–432.

09340   MARCH, H.
Zweierlei Mass. [*Two Criteria*]. In March, H. (ed.), Verfolgung Und
Angst. Stuttgart: Ernst Klett Verlag, 1960, 148–157.

09350   MARCH, H.
Verfolgung Und Angst. In Ihren Leib-Seelischen Auswirkungen.
[*Persecution and Anxiety*]. By: Bayer and Kisker, Cremerius, March,
Strauss. Stuttgart: Ernst Klett Verlag, 1960.

09360   MARCH, H.
Die Bedeutung Der Anamnese In Der Gutachterpraxis. [*The
Importance of the Anamnesis in the Expert Statements*]. In March, H.
(ed.), Verfolgung Und Angst. Stuttgart: Ernst Klett Verlag, 1960,
130–147.

09370   MARCH, H.
Die Schicksale Zweier Juden Und Ein Beispielgutachten. [*The Fate of
Two Jews and an Example of an Expert Statement*]. In March, H. (ed.),
Verfolgung Und Angst. Stuttgart: Ernst Klett Verlag, 1960, 158–191.

09380   MARCH, H.
(Ed.), Medizin und Menschlichkeit. [*Medicine and Humanity*].
Herford: Nicholaische Verlagsbuchhandlung 1968.

09390   MARCUS, S.
Study Carried Out in England on a Group of 300 Young Refugees. In
Later Effects of Imprisonment and Deportation. International
Conference Organized by the World Veterans Federation. The Hague:
World Veterans Federation, 1961, 158–159.

09400   MARCUS, P.
Jewish Consciousness after the Holocaust. In Luel, S. A. and P. Marcus
(eds.), Psychoanalytic Reflections on the Holocaust: Selected Essays.
New York: Ktav Publishing House, 1984, 179–198.

09410   MARIN, B.
A Post-Holocaust "Anti-Semitism without Anti-Semites?" Austria as a
Case in Point. Polit Psych (1980) 2(2):57–74.

09420   MARTINO, C.; SCIARRA, M. A.
Psycho-Pathologische Und Gerichtsmedizinische Erwägungen Über
Die Chronischen Reaktionsdepressionen Bei Ehemaligen Internierten,
Deportierten, Etc. [Psychopathological and Forensic Discussions on
the Chronic Reactive Depression in Ex-Deportees and Prisoners]. In
Ätio-Pathogenese Und Therapie Der Erschöpfung Und Vorzeitigen
Vergreisung. IV Internationaler Medizinischer Kongress Der F.I.R.
Bucharest: Verlag Der F.I.R., 1964, 344–350.

09430   MASLOWSKI, J.
[30th Anniversary of the Liberation of the Auschwitz Camp.
Commemorative Services Organized by the Cracow Medical Society].
Przeglad Lekarski (1976) 33(1):200–212.

09440   MASLOWSKI, J.
Okupacyjna Tematyka Lekarska W Polskich Publikacjach Z Roku
1977. [Medical Problems Relating to the Nazi Occupation Described in
Polish Publications in 1977]. Przeglad Lekarski (1978) 35(1):237–253.

09450   MASLOWSKI, J.
[Letters Written to the Periodical "Auschwitz," Published by the Medical
Review]. Przeglad Lekarski (1979) 36(1):229–235.

09460   MASLOWSKI, J.
[Medical Subjects Relating to Nazi Occupation in Polish Publications in
1979]. Przeglad Lekarski (1980) 37(1):213–218.

09470   MASLOWSKI, J.; PARYSKI, E. R.; KURGAN, A.; MICHALSKI, E.
Contents of Preceding Issues of "Przeglad Lekarski" (Medical Review)
Devoted to Medical Problems of the Period of Nazi Occupation (author's
translation)]. Przeglad Lekarski (1981) 38(1):249–269.

09480   MASLOWSKI, J.
[Medical Topics Dealing with the German Occupation in Polish Works
Published in 1980]. Przeglad Lekarski (1981) 38(1):229–248.

09490   MASLOWSKI, J.
[Letters Written to the "Przeglad Lekarski" (Medical Review) on the
Subject of Auschwitz (III)]. Przeglad Lekarski (1981) 38(1):216–220.

09500   MASLOWSKI, J.
[35th Anniversary of the Liberation of Auschwitz Memorialized at the
Cracow Medical Society]. Przeglad Lekarski (1981) 38(1):210–215.

09510   MASLOWSKI, J.
[Antoni Kepinski during the Years 1939–1947]. Przeglad Lekarski
(1981) 38(1):126–137.

09520   MASLOWSKI, J.
[The Subject of Medicine during the Occupation in Polish Publications
of the Year 1983]. Przeglad Lekarski (1984) 41(1):159–177.

09530   MATUSSEK, P.
Die Konzentrationslagerhaft Als Belastungssituation. [*Imprisonment in Concentration Camps as a Stress Situation*]. Nervenarzt (1961) 32:538–542.

09540   MATUSSEK, P.
Die Rückgliederung Von Verfolgten Die Bewältigung Ihres Schicksals. [*Rehabilitation of Persecutees Coping With Their Fate*]. Therapiewoche (1963) 1109–1113.

09550   MATUSSEK, P.
Spätfolgen Bei KZ-Haeftlingen. [*Late Effects in Concentration Camp Prisoners*]. Bild Der Wissenschaft (1969) 803–809.

09560   MATUSSEK, P.
Psychoreaktive Störungen Bei Ehemaligen KZ-Häftlingen. [*Psychoreactive Disturbances in Ex-Concentration Camp Prisoners*]. In Herberg, H.J. (ed.), Spätschäden Nach Extremebelastungen. II Internationalen Medizinisch-Juristischen Konferenz in Düsseldorf, 1969. Herford: Nicholaische Verlagsbuchhandlung, 1971, 182–186.

09570   MATUSSEK, P.
Die Konzentrationslagerhaft Und Ihre Folgen. [*Internment in Concentration Camps and Its Consequences*]. Berlin: Springer Verlag, (1971). Psychiatry Series, Part II With Grigat, Haiböck, Halbach, Kemmler, Mantell, Triebel, Vardy, Wedel. English translation, 1975.

09580   MATUSSEK, P.
Late Symptomatology among Former Concentration Camp Inmates. In Arieti, S. (ed.), The World Biennial of Psychiatry and Psychotherapy. New York: Basic Books, 1971.

09590   MATUSSEK, P.; GRIGAT, R.; HAIBOCK, H.; HALBACH, G.
Late Effects of Concentration Camp Stress. IRCS (1973) 39-7-2 (International Research Communication System).

09600   MATUSSEK, P.
Psychische Schäden Bei Konzentrationslagerhäftlingen. [*Psychic Disturbances in Concentration Camp Prisoners*]. In Psychiatrie Der Gegenwart. Berlin, Heidelberg: Springer Verlag, 1975, 387–427.

09610   MATUSSEK, P.
Dimensionen Psychischer Stoerungen Als Spätfolge Bei Ehemaligen KZ Häftlingen. Eine Faktorenanalytische Untersuchung. [*Dimension of Psychic Disturbances in Ex-Concentration Camp Prisoners. An Investigation Based on Factorial Analysis*]. VI Internationaler Medizinischer Kongress Der F.I.R., Prague, 1976.

09620   MATUSSEK, P.
Bedrängnis Und Bewältigung Im Spiegel Des Einzelschicksals. Individuelle Stressreaktion Bei Ehemaligen KZ Häftlingen. [*Stress and Coping as Seen in Individual Fates. Individual Stress Reactions in Ex-Concentration Camp Prisoners*]. Klinische Wochenschrift (1977) 55:869–876.

09630 MAZIARSKI, S.
[*From Cracow to Sachsenhausen*]. Przeglad Lekarski (1981)
38(1):143–151.

09640 MEADOW, D. A.
*The Preparatory Interview: A Client-Focused Approach with Children of
Holocaust Survivors.* Social Work with Groups (1981)
4(3–4):135–144.

09650 MEERLOO, J. A. M.
*Neurologism and Denial of Psychic Trauma in Extermination Camp
Survivors.* Am J Psychiat (1963) 120:65–66. Also in Krystal, H. (ed.),
Massive Psychic Trauma. New York: International Universities Press,
1968, 72–75.

09660 MEERLOO, J. A. M.
Delayed Mourning in Victims of Extermination Camps. J Hillside
Hospital (1963) 12:96–98. Also in Krystal, H. (ed.), Massive Psychic
Trauma. New York: International Universities Press, 1968, 70–72.

09670 MEERLOO, J. A. M.
*Persecution Trauma and the Reconditioning of Emotional Life: A Brief
Survey.* Am J Psychiat (1969) 125(9):1187–1191.

09680 MEERLOO, J. A. M.
Hoe het concentratiekamp zijn slachtoffers programmeert. [*How the
Concentration Camp Programmes Its Victims*]. Arts Wereld (1975)
8:14–32.

09690 MEIJERING, W. L.
Die Behandlung Ehemaliger Widerstands-Kämpfer Und Opfer
Nazistischer Und Japaniche Verfolgung Der Niederländer. [*The
Treatment in the Netherlands of Ex-Underground Fighters and Victims
of Nazi and Japanese Persecution*]. 1977. Manuscript.

09700 MELTZER, D.
Terror, Persecution, Dread—A Dissection of Paranoid Anxieties.
Internat J Psycho-Anal (1968) 49:396–401.

09710 MELVILLE, J.
The Scars of the Survivors. New Society (1979) 3:15–18.

09720 MENDE, W.
Grenzen Der Seelischen Belastbarkeit. [*The Limits of Psychological
Tolerance*]. Med Klin (1962) 57:1636–1640.

09730 MENDE, W.
Gutachterliche Probleme Bei Der Beurteilung Erlebnisreaktiver
Schädigungen. [*Problems of Expert Evaluation in Cases of
Traumatization Caused by Life Events*]. In Paul, H. and H. J. Herberg
(eds.), Psychische Spätschäden Nach Politischer Verfolgung. Basel: S.
Karger 1963, 281–292.

09740 MENDE, W.
Begutachtungsfragen bei Erlebnisreaktiven Störungen. [*Problems of*

Expert Evaluation of Disturbances due to Life Events]. In Herberg, H.J.
(ed.), Spätschäden Nach Extremebelastungen. II Internationalen
Medizinisch-Juristischen Konferenz in Duesseldorf (1969). Herford:
Nicholaische Verlagsbuchhandlung 1971, 190–192.

09750   MENKE, J.
Die Soziale Integration Jüdischer Flüchtlinge Des Ehemaligen
Regierungslagers "Foehrenwald" in Den Drei Westdeutschen
Grosstädten Düsseldorf, Frankfurt and München [*The Social
Integration of Former Jewish Refugees from Government Camps
"Foehrenwald" in Three West German Cities, Dusseldorf, Frankfurt and
Munich*]. Bielefeld: Bertelsmann, 1960.

09760   MEROWITZ, M.
*The Aging Survivor of the Holocaust. Words before We Go: The
Experience of Holocaust and Its Effect on Communication in the Aging
Survivor.* J Geri Psychiat (1981) 14(2):241–244.

09770   MEYER, J.
Die Abnormalen Erlebnisreaktionen Im Kriege Bei Truppe und
Zivilbevölkerung. [*The Abnormal Experience and Reactions in War by
Soldiers and the Civilian Population.*] In H. Gruhle (ed.), Psychiatrie
der Gegenwart, Vol. 3. Berlin: Springer, 1961.

09780   MEYEROWITZ, H.
Case Work Services for Adolescent Newcomers. Jewish Soc Serv Q
(1947) 24:136–146.

09790   MEYROUNE, C.
Die Bedeutung Der Aufstellung Periodischer Gesundheitsbilanzen Für
Die Bekämpfung Des Corzeitigen Alterns. [*The Importance of
Periodical Health Controls in the Combat against Premature Aging*]. In
Die Behandlung Der Asthenie Und Der Vorzeitigen Vergreisung Bei
Ehmaligen Widerstanskämpfern Und KZ Haeftlingen. III
Internationale Medizinische Konferenz. Luettich: Verlag Der F.I.R.,
1961, 242–254.

09800   MICHEL, M.
Spätschäden Und Summationsschäden. [*Late and Summation
Sequelae*]. In Michel, M. (ed.), Gesundheitsschäden Durch Verfolgung
Und Gefangenschaft Und Ihre Spätfolgen. Frankfurt Am Main:
Röderberg Verlag, 1955, 48–51.

09810   MICHEL, M.
Gesundheitsschäden Durch Verfolgung Und Gedangenschaft Und Ihre
Spätfolgen. [*Disturbances of Health Caused by Persecution and
Imprisonment and Their Late Sequels*]. Frankfurt Am Main: Röderberg
Verlag, 1955. With papers by Canivet, Deveen, Fog, Mogens, Hagen,
Helweg, Hermann, Hoffmeyer, Kieler, Munke, Thaysen, E.H.
Thygesen, Thaysen, J.H. Targowla, Dupont, Fichez, Gilbert-Dreyfus,
Worms, Desoille, Richet, Blockhin, Reid.

09820   MICHEL, M.
Einige Probleme Der Begutachtung Von Verfolgungsschäden

Deutscher Opfer Des Nazi-Regimes. [*Some Problems of the Evaluation of Persecution-Caused Disturbances in German Victims of the Nazi Regime*]. In Michel, M. (ed.), Gesundheitsschäden Durch Verfolgung Und Gefdangenschaft Und Ihre Spätfolgen. Frankfurt Am Main: Röderberg Verlag, 1955, 297–316.

09830   MILCINSKI, J.
Crisis in Medical Ethics. In Auschwitz, Inhuman Medicine, Anthology, Vol. 1, Part 1. Warsaw: International Auschwitz Committee, 1970, 123–146.

09840   MILIKOWSKI, H.
Het KZ-Syndroom en de Psychiatrische Mythen. [*The Concentration Camp Syndrome and the Psychiatric Myths*]. In H. Milikowski, Sociologie als verzet, over KZ-syndroom, gezinsproblemen, sociale en seksuele relaties en agressie. Amsterdam: Van Gennep 1973, 87–122.

09850   MILIKOWSKI, H.
Daarom wil ik pleiten voor verzetstherapie. [*Therefore I wish to Plead for Resistance Therapy*]. In H. Milikowski, Sociologie als verzet, over KZ-syndroom, gezinsproblemen, sociale en seksuele relaties en agressie. Amsterdam: Van Gennep 1973, 141–149.

09860   MILLER, L.
Social Roots of Persecution. Israel-Netherlands Symposium on the Impact of Persecution. 2, Dalfsen, Amsterdam, 14–18 April 1980. The Netherlands: Rijswijk, 1981, 21–26.

09870   MINKOWSKI, E.
L'Anesthésie Affective. [*The Affective Anesthesia*]. Ann Méd Psychol (1946) 104:80–88.

09880   MINKOWSKI, E.
Les Conséquences Psychologiques et Psychopathologiques de la Guerre et du Nazisme. [*The Psychologic and Psychopathologic Consequences of War and Nazism*]. Schw Arch (1947) 61:280.

09890   MISCHEL, E.
Personal Reflections on the Holocaust and Holocaust Survivors. Am J Psychoanal (1979) 39(4):369–376.

09900   MITSCHERLICH, A.; MIELKE, F.
Doctors of Infamy. The Story of Nazi Medical Crimes. New York: Henry Schuman, 1949.

09910   MITSCHERLICH, A.; MITSCHERLICH, M.
The Inability to Mourn. New York: Grove Press, 1975.

09920   MITSCHERLICH, A.
Die Vorurteilskrankheit. [*The Sickness of Prejudice*]. Psyche (1962/63) 16:241

09930   MITSCHERLICH-NIELSEN, M.
[*The Past within the Present. On the Film "Playing for Time"*]. Psyche (1981) 35(7):611-615.

09940   MOCK-DEGEN, M.
De ethische aspekten van een psychiatrisch onderzoek,
kanttekeningen bij het proefschrift over de Joodse oorlogswezen. [*The
Ethical Aspects of a Psychiatric Research, Margin Notes on a Proof
Manuscript Concerning Jewish War Foster Children*]. Maandblad
Geestelijke Volksgezondheid (1980) 35(4):290–301.

09950   MOLLHAFF, G.
[*About Insurance Medical Evaluation of Psychoreactive Disturbances
(Author's Translation)*]. Rechtsmed (1975) 46(6):291–296.

09960   MONNICKENDAM, M.
*Formal Non-Material Services for the Traumatized and the Social
Setting in Israel.* Israel-Netherlands Symposium on the Impact of
Persecution. 2, Dalfsen, Amsterdam, 14–18 April 1980. The
Netherlands: Rijswijk, 1981, 43–46.

09970   MORIC-PETROVIC, S.
*Neuropsychiatric After Effects on a Group of Participants in the
People's Liberation War of Yugoslavia.* In Later Effects of
Imprisonment and Deportation. International Conference Organized
by the World Veterans Federation. The Hague: World Veterans
Federation, 1961, 96–99.

09980   MOROSOW, V.M.
Late Sequelae in Former Deportees and Concentration Camp Survivors.
J Neuropathol and Psychiat (1958) 58(3):373–380.

09990   MORSE, D.O.
*Studying the Holocaust and Human Behavior: Effects on Early
Adolescent Self-Esteem, Locus of Control, Acceptance of Self and Others,
and Philosophy of Human Nature.* Ph.D. diss., California School of
Professional Psychology, Fresno, 1981. page 4209 in Vol 42/10-B of
Dissertation Abstracts International. Order No: AAD82-04014.

10000   MOSES, R.
A Fifty Year Span: Some Reflections on Israelis and Germans. Isr J
Psychiat Rel Sci (1983) 20(1–2):155–167.

10010   MOSES, R.
An Israeli Psychoanalyst Looks Back in 1983. In Luel, S.A. and P.
Marcus (eds.), Psychoanalytic Reflections on the Holocaust: Selected
Essays. New York: Ktav Publishing House, 1984, 53–70.

10020   MOSKOVITZ, S.
*Love Despite Hate. Child Survivors of The Holocaust and Their Adult
Lives.* New York: Schocken, 1982.

10021   MOSKOVITZ, S.
Longitudinal Follow Up of Child Survivors. Presented at the APA
Symposium on Child Survivors of the Holocaust—40 Years Later.
Los Angeles 1984. In J Amer Acad Child Psychiat, July 1985.

10030   MOSKA, D.
[*Concentration Camps for Polish Nationals in Upper Silesia*]. Przeglad
Lekarski (1974) 31(1):134–139.

10040   MOST, Van der, M.; RAVENSTEIJN, Van, L.;
        WILBAUT-GUILONARD, T.
        De Tweede Generatie. [*The Second Generation*]. Maandblad
        Geestelijke Volksgezondheid (1973) 28:227–231.

10050   MOSTYSSER, T.
        Growing Up in America with a Holocaust Heritage. Jewish Digest
        (1975) 21:3–6.

10060   MOSTYSSER, T.
        The Weight of the Past: Reminiscences of a Survivor's Child. In
        Steinitz, L. (ed.), Living after the Holocaust: Reflections by the
        Post-War Generation in America. New York: Bloch, 1975, 3–21.

10070   MOYNIER, G.
        Studie Über Die Folgen Organischer Störungen, Infolge Des Lebens
        In Der Illigalitaet. [*Study on the Sequels of Organic Disturbances
        Caused by Life in Illegality*]. In Ätio-Pathogenese Und Therapie Der
        Erschöpfung Und Vorzeitigen Vergreisung. IV Internationaler
        Medizinischer Kongress Der F.I.R. Bucharest: Verlag Der F.I.R., 1964,
        88–89.

10080   MUELLER-HEGEMANN, D.
        Zur Therapie Neurotischer Folgezustände Nach Faschistischer Haft.
        [*The Therapy of Neurotic Sequelae after Fascist Imprisonment*]. In Die
        Behandlung Der Asthenie Und Der Vorzeitigen Vergreisung Bei
        Ehemaligen Widerstanskämpfern Und KZ Häftlingen. III
        International Medizinische Konferenz. Luettich: Verlag Der F.I.R.,
        1961, 77–79.

10090   MUELLER-HEGEMANN, D.; SPITZNER, G.
        Reihenuntersuchungen Bei Verfolgten Des Naziregimes-Mit
        Besondere Berücksichtigung Von Einzelhaftfolgen. [*Serial
        Investigations of Persecutees of the Nazi Regime with Special Regard to
        the Sequelae of Isolation*]. Deutsche Gesundheitswesen (1963)
        18:107–116.

10100   MUELLER-HEGEMANN, D.
        Erfahrungen Auf Dem Gebiete Der Begutachtung Und Rehabilitation
        Von Verfolgten Des Naziregimes. [*Evaluation and Rehabilitation of
        Persecutees of the Nazi Regime*]. In Ätio-Pathogenese Und Therapie
        Der Erschöpfung Und Vorzeitigen Vergreisung. IV Internationaler
        Medizinischer Kongress Der F.I.R. Bucharest: Verlag Der F.I.R., 1964,
        66–72.

10110   MUELLER-HEGEMANN, D.
        Über Schaedigungen Und Störungen Des Nervensystems Bei
        Verfolgten Des Naziregimes (VDN) Und Deren Begutachtung.
        [*Traumatizations of the Nervous Systems in Persecutees of the Nazi
        Regime and Their Evaluation*]. Deutsche Gesundheitswesen (1966)
        21:561–568.

10120   MULDER, D.
        The Uselessness of General Diagnostic Concepts. In Ayalon, O. (ed.) The
        Holocaust and Its Perseverance. Assen 1983, Holland, 17–24.

10130   MURY, L.
Untersuchungen Psychischer Und Psychosomatischer Störungen Bei
Ehemaligen Konzentrationslagerhäftlingen 23 Jahre Nach Der
Befreiung. [*Investigations of Psychic and Psychosomatic Disturbances
in Ex-Concentration Camp Prisoners, 23 Years after the Liberation*]. In
Ermüdung Und Vorzeitiges Altern. Folge Von Extremebelastungen. V
Internationaler Medizinischer Kongress Der F.I.R., Paris, 1970,
Leipzig: Johann Ambrosius, 1973, 215–242.

10140   MUSAPH, H.
Post Concentratiekampsyndroom. [*The Post Concentration Camp
Syndrome*]. Maandblad Geestelijke Volksgezondheid (1973) 28,
207–217.

10150   MUSAPH, H.
The Second Generation of War Victims: Psychopathological Problems.
Isr J Psychiat Rel Sci (1981) 18(1):3–14.

10160   MUSAPH, H.
De opvoeders van de tweede generatie. [*The Educators of the Second
Generation*]. In Psycho-sociale problematiek van de tweede generatie
(2), *(Psycho-social Problems of the Second Generation)*, een bundeling
van de drie inleidingen gehouden op de studiedag over de
psycho-sociale problematiek van de tweede generatie georganiseerd
door de Stichting ICODO op 9 juni 1983. Utrecht, 1983, 5–10.

10170   NADEL, C.; VOLLHARDT, B.
Coping with Illness by a Concentration Camp Survivor. Gen Hosp
Psychiat (1979) (2):175–181.

10180   NAGY, Z.; COCHYANOVA, B.; BALAZ, V.
Gezielte Sozial-Medizinische Studie Unter Teilnehmern Des
Widerstandskämpfes Und Ihre Dynamischen Elemente. [*Specific
Socio-Medical Study of Resistance Fighters and its Dynamic Elements*].
VI Internationaler Medizinischer Kongress Der F.I.R., Prague, 1976.

10190   NATHAN, T. S.; EITINGER, L.; WINNIK, H. Z.
*A Psychiatric Study of Survivors of the Nazi Holocaust. A Study of
Hospitalized Patients.* Isr Ann Psychiat Rel Disc (1964) 2(1):47–80.

10200   NATHAN, T. S.
Hapsikhodinamikah Shel Hafra'ot Betifkud Yots'ei Hashoah
Kehorim. [*The Psychodynamics of Disturbances in Parental
Functioning of Holocaust Survivors*]. Presented at the Eleventh Israel
Neuropsychiatric Congress, 1969, Haifa. Manuscript.

10210   NATHAN, T. S.
Disturbed Parent Role in Holocaust Survivors. Isr Ann Psychiat (1969)
8:234.

10220   NATHAN, T. S.
*Research Proposal on the Parent-Child Relationship in the Holocaust
Survivors in Kibbutz and Urban Society.* Jerusalem, 1973. Manuscript.

10230   NATHAN, T. S.
Children of Holocaust Survivors—A Clinical Study. 8th International

Congress of the International Association for Child Psychiatry and Allied Professions, "The Vulnerable Child," Philadelphia, 1974.

10240 NATHAN, T. S.
Dor Sheny Lenitzoley Hashoa Bemechkarim Psychosocialiim. [*The Second Generation of Holocaust Survivors in Psychosocial Research*]. In Studies of the Holocaust Period, Vol. 2. Tel Aviv. Hakibutz Hameuchad Publishing House, 1981, 13–26.

10250 NELKIN, M.
Survivors of Nazi Concentration Camps: Psychopathology and Views of Psychotherapy. Can J Psychiat Nurs (1979) 20(6):560–568.

10260 NEMETH, M.C.
Psychosis in a Concentration Camp Survivor, A Case Presentation. Int Psychiat Clin (1971) 8:135–146.

10270 NETTER, A.
On the Physiopathology of Amenorrhea in Concentration Camps. In Later Effects of Imprisonment and Deportation. International Conference Organized by the World Veterans Federation. The Hague: World Veterans Federation, 1961, 73–77.

10280 NEURATH, P.M.
Social Life in the German Concentration Camps Dachau and Buchenwald. Ph.D. diss., Columbia University, 1951. Page 111 in Vol 12/01 of Dissertation Abstracts International. Order No: AAD00-03372.

10290 NEWMAN, L.
Emotional Disturbance in Children of Holocaust Survivors. Social Casework (1979) 43–50.

10300 NIEDERLAND, W.G.
Discussion of K. Hoppe. *The Psychodynamics of Concentration Camp Victims.* Psychoanal For (1960) 1:80.

10310 NIEDERLAND, W.G.
The Problem of the Survivor. The Psychiatric Evaluation of Emotional Disorders in Survivors of Nazi Persecution. J Hillside Hosp (1961) 10:233–247. Also in Krystal, H. (ed.), Massive Psychic Trauma. New York: International Universities Press, 1968, 8–22.

10320 NIEDERLAND, W.G.
Psychiatric Disorders among Persecution Victims. A Contribution to the Understanding of Concentration Camp Pathology and its After-Effects. J Nerv Ment Dis (1964) 139:458–474.

10330 NIEDERLAND, W.G.
Ein Blick In Die Tiefen Der "Unbewältigten Vergangenheit Gegenwart." [*A Look in Depth at the Past and Present*]. Psyche (1966) 20:466.

10340 NIEDERLAND, W.G.
The Second Wayne State University Workshop on the Late Sequels of Massive Psychic Traumatization. Papers published in Krystal, H. (ed.),

Massive Psychic Trauma. New York: International Universities Press, 1968.

10350 NIEDERLAND, W. G.
Clinical Observations on the "Survivor Syndrome." Int J Psycho-Anal (1968) 49:313–315.

10360 NIEDERLAND, W. G.; KRYSTAL, H.
Clinical Observations on the "Survivor" Syndrome. In Krystal, H. (ed.), Massive Psychic Trauma. New York: International Universities Press, 1968, 327–348.

10370 NIEDERLAND, W. G.
An Interpretation of the Psychological Stresses and Defenses in Concentration Camp Life and the Late After-Effects. In Krystal, H. (ed.), Massive Psychic Trauma. New York: International Universities Press, 1968, 60–70.

10380 NIEDERLAND, W. G.
The Psychiatric Evaluation of Emotional Disorders in Survivors of Nazi Persecution. In Krystal, H. (ed.), Massive Psychic Trauma. New York: International Universities Press, 1968, 8–22.

10400 NIEDERLAND, W. G.
Introducing Notes on the Concept, Definition and Range of Psychiatric Trauma. Int Psychiat Clin (1971) 8:1. Also in Krystal, H. and G. Niederland (eds.), Psychic Traumatization. Boston: Little, Brown, 1971, 1–9.

10410 NIEDERLAND, W. G.
Clinical Observations on the Survivor Syndrome. In Parker, R. S. (ed.), The Emotional Stress of War, Violence, and Peace. Pittsburgh: Stanwix House, 1972.

10420 NIEDERLAND, W. G.
The Survivor Syndrome: Further Observations and Dimensions. J Amer Psychoanal Ass (1981) 29:413–425.

10430 NIEDOJADLO, E.
The Camp "Hospital" in Buna. In Auschwitz, In Hell They Preserved Human Dignity, Anthology, Vol. 2, Part 2. Warsaw: International Auschwitz Committee, 1971, 46–57.

10440 NIELSEN, H.
[*Disability during the Years 1946–1979 among Members of the Danish Resistance Movement Deported to German Concentration Camps*]. Ugeskr Laeger (1983) 145(5):350–355.

10450 NIELSEN, H.
[*1943–1979 Mortality among Members of the Danish Resistance Movement Deported to German Concentration Camps*]. Ugeskr Laeger (1983) 145(5):345–350.

10460 NIELSEN, H.
[*Disability and Its Course during the Years 1946–1979 Among*

Concentration Camp Prisoners Previously Exposed to Severe Stress].
Ugeskr Laeger (1983) 145(12):935–940.

10470 NIELSEN, H.; MADSEN, M.
[*The Significance of the Strain of Deportation and the Occupation for
the Postwar Mortality and Disability of Surviving Concentration Camp
Prisoners*]. Ugeskr Laeger (1983) 145(12):929–934.

10480 NIEWIAROWICZ, R.
[*Reminiscences about Kotarbinski, Physician and Concentration Camp
Prisoners*]. Przeglad Lekarski (1970) 26(1):266–270.

10490 NIEWIAROWICZ, R.
[*Medicine in Articulo Mortis in Nazi Prisons and Concentration
Camps*]. Przeglad Lekarski (1973) 30(1):179–188.

10500 NIKOLIC, D.
*Epidemiological Table of Tuberculosis among Internees and the
Consequences of Tuberculosis.* In Later Effects of Imprisonment and
Deportation. International Conference Organized by the World
Veterans Federation. The Hague: World Veterans Federation, 1961,
67–68.

10510 NIKOLIC, D.
Les Conséquences Tardives de la Tuberculose chez les Déportés dans
les Camps de Concentration Pendant le Deuxième Guerre Mondiale.
[*Late Sequels of Tuberculosis among the Deportees in the Concentration
Camps During World War II*]. VI Congrès Médical International de la
F.I.R., Prague, 1976.

10520 NIREMBERSKI, M.
Psychological Investigation of a Group of Internees at Belsen-Camp. J
Men Sci (1946) 92:60–74.

10530 NISSIM, L.; BENEDETTI, L.; PERRETTA, G.
Soziale Neu-Eingliederung In Italien (Nazi Und Faschistenopfer).
[*Social Rehabilitation in Italy (Victims of Nazis and Fascists)*]. In
Michel, M. (ed.), Gesundheitsschaeden Durch Verfolgung Und
Gefangenschaft Und Ihre Spätfolgen. Frankfurt Am Main: Röderberg
Verlag, 1955, 238–239.

10540 NOORDHOEK-HEGT, W.G.
Die Situation In Den Niederlanden. [*The Situation in the
Netherlands*]. In Herberg, H.J.(ed.), Die Beurteilung Von
Gesundheitsschäden Nach Gefangenschaft Und Verfolgung.
Internationalen Medizinisch-Juristischen Symposiums in Köln (1967).
Herford: Nicholaische Verlagsbuchhandlung, 1967, 29–33.

10550 NOWAK, J.A.
Die Problematik Des KZ Syndroms Und Eigene
Behandlungsmethoden Und Erfolge. [*Problems of the Concentration
Camp Syndrome and Personal Methods of Treatment and Results*]. VI
Internationaler Medizinischer Kongress Der F.I.R., Paris, 1970.
Leipzig: Johann Ambrosius, 1973, 376–386.

10560   NOWAK, J. A.
Verbrechen An Kindern Und Jugendlichen Während Der Nazi
Okkupationszeit. [Crimes on Children and Adolescents during the Nazi
Occupation]. In Ermuedung Und Vorzeitiges Altern. Folg Von
Extremebelastungen. V Internationaler Medizinischer Kongress Der
F.I.R., Paris, 1970. Leipzig: Johann Ambrosius, 1973, 376– 386.

10570   NOWAK, J. A.
Die Problematik Des KZ Syndroms Und Eigene
Behandlungsmethoden Und Erfolge. [Problems of the Concentration
Camp Syndrome and Personal Methods of Treatment and Results]. VI
Internationaler Medizinischer Kongress Der F.I.R., Prague, 1976.

10580   NOWAKOWSKA, M. L.
"Infirmerie des Femmes" à Birkenau. [The Women's Sick Bay in
Birkenau]. Cahier d'inf F.I.R. (1975) 6:1– 4.

10590   NOWICKI, J.
[After the Liberation of the Sandbostel Camp]. Przeglad Lekarski (1975)
32(1):182– 187.

10600   NOWOSIELSKI, A.
[At the Neuengamme Concentration Camp. Dr. Zyman Szafraski].
Przeglad Lekarski (1977) 34(1):207– 211.

10610   OFMAN, J.
Separation-Individuation in Children of Nazi Holocaust Survivors and
Its Relationship to Perceived Parental Overvaluation. Ph.D. diss.,
California School of Professional Psychology, Berkeley, 1981. Page
3434 in Vol 42/08-B of Dissertation Abstracts International. Order
No: AAD82-01496.

10620   OLBRYCHT, J.
Das Nazistische Sanitätspersonal Führte Eine Aktive
Zusammenarbeit Mit der S.S.—Verwaltung von Auschwitz. [The Nazi
Health Office Actively Participated with the SS Administration in
Auschwitz]. In Auschwitz, Inhuman Medicine, Anthology, Vol. 1, Part
1. Warsaw: International Auschwitz Committee, 1970, 147– 205.

10630   OLINER, M. M.
Hysterical Features among Children of Survivors. In Bergmann, M. S.
and M. E. Jucovy (eds.), Generations of the Holocaust. New York:
Basic Books, 1982, 267– 286.

10640   OLSZYNA, R.
[Preliminary List of Physicians at the Gross-Rosen Concentration
Camp]. Przeglad Lekarski (1970) 26(1):169– 171.

10650   ORNSTEIN, A.
The Aging Survivor of the Holocaust. The Effects of the Holocaust on
Life-Cycle Experiences: The Creation and Recreation of Families. J Geri
Psychiat (1981) 14(2):135– 154.

10660   ORWID, M.; SZYMUSIK, A.; TEUTSCH, A.
Purpose and Method of Psychiatric Examinations of Former Prisoners

of the Auschwitz Concentration Camp. In Auschwitz, It Did Not End in Forty-Five, Anthology, Vol. 3, Part 2. Warsaw: International Auschwitz Committee, 1972, 130–142.

10670 ORWID, M.
Socio-Psychiatric Consequences of the Stay in the Concentration Camp Auschwitz-Birkenau. in Auschwitz, It Did Not End in Forty-Five, Anthology, Vol. 3, Part 3. Warsaw: International Auschwitz Committee, 1972, 174–206.

10680 OSTWALD, P.F.; BITTNER, E.
Life Adjustment after Severe Persecution. Am J Psychiat (1968) 124:1393–1400.

10690 OSTWALD, P.T.
Studies of Concentration Camp Victims. Prepared for Symposium on Stress. Tel Aviv, 1972. Manuscript.

10700 OSVIK, K.
Internal Medical Findings in Ex-Concentration Camp Inmates. In Later Effects of Imprisonment and Deportation. International Conference Organized by the World Veterans Federation. The Hague: World Veterans Federation, 1961, 122–123.

10710 OSVIK, K.
Indremedisinske Funn Hos Tidligere Konsentrasjons-Leirfanger. [*Internal Medical Findings in Ex-Concentration Camp Prisoners*]. Undersoekelse Av Norske Tidligere Konsentrasjonsleirfanger. In Tidsskr Norske Laegeforening (1961) 81:811–812.

10720 OYEN, O.
Die Situation in Norwegen. [*The Situation in Norway*]. In Herberg, H.J. (ed.), Die Beurteilung Von Gesundheitsschäden Nach Gefdangenschaft Und Verfolgung. Internationalen Medizinisch-Juristischen Symposiums in Köln, 1967. Herford: Nicholaische Verlagsbuchhandlung, 1967, 44–45.

10730 PACZULA, T.
The Organization and Administration of the Camp Hospital in the Concentration Camp Auschwitz 1. In Auschwitz, In Hell They Preserved Human Dignity, Anthology, Vol. 2, Part 1. Warsaw, 1971, 38–75.

10740 PALMBLAD, J.; LEVI, L.; BURGER, A.; MELANDER, A.; WESTGREN, U.; SCHENCK, H. Von; SKUDE, G.
Effects of Total Energy Withdrawal (Fasting) on the Levels of Growth Hormone, Thyrotropin, Cortisol, Adrenaline, Noradrenaline, T4, T3, and RT3 in Healthy Males. Reports from the Laboratory for Clinical Stress Research (1976) 47:1–27.

10750 PANASEWICZ, J.; LUCKIEWICZ, B.
Folgen Des Konzentrationslager Hungerdystrophiesyndroms Unter Besonderer Berücksichtigung Hämotologischer Strörungen. [*Consequences of the Concentration Camp Dystrophia of Inanition-Syndrome with Special Regard to Haematological Diseases*].

In Ermüdung Und Vorzeitiges Altern. Folge Von
Extremebelastungen. V Internationalen Medizinischer Kongress Der
F.I.R. Paris, 1970. Leipzig: Johann Ambrosius, 1973, 56–71.

10760   PARKER, F.K.
*Dominant Attitudes of Adult Children of Holocaust Survivors toward
Their Parents.* Ph.D. diss., Saybrook Institute, 1983. Page 2230 in Vol
44/07-B of Dissertation Abstracts International. Order No:
AAD83-25704.

10770   PATON, A.
Mission to Belsen 1945. Br Med J [Clin Res] (1981)
19:283(6307):1656–1659.

10780   PATTI, M.
Les Facteurs Psychoaffectiés dans la Determination du Syndrome
Psychosomatique de la Deportation et dans L'Instauration de la
Psychose Chronique Ainsi Dite "De Ronce Artificielle." [*The
Psychoaffective Factors in Psychosomatic Syndromes Caused by
Deportation and in Chronic Psychoses, the So-Called "De Ronce
Artificielle"*]. Ann Med Di Navale (1964) 69:501–506.

10790   PATTISON, E.M.
*The Holocaust as Sin: Requirements in Psychoanalytic Theory for
Human Evil and Mature Morality.* In Luel, S.A. and P. Marcus (eds.),
Psychoanalytic Reflections on the Holocaust: Selected Essays. New
York: Ktav Publishing House, 1984, 71–91.

10800   PAUL, H.A.
Der Mechanismus Einer Flucht In Die Dystrophie. [*The Mechanism of
a "Flight Into Dystrophy"*]. Zeitschr Psychother Med Psychol (1957)
(6)7:249–257.

10810   PAUL, H.A.
Über Den Psycho-Stress. [*On the Psycho-Stress*]. Psychol Prax (1958)
1:1–13.

10820   PAUL, H.A.
Charakterveränderungen Durch Kriegsgefangenschaft Und
Dystrophie. [*Changes of Character by War Imprisonment and
Dystrophy*]. In Extreme Lebensverhältnisse Und Ihre Folgen. Bericht
Über Den 4 Ärztekongress Für Pathologie, Therapie Und
Begutachtung Der Heimkehrerkrankheiten in Düsseldorf, 1959, Band
8, 41–54.

10830   PAUL, H.A.
Bemerkungen Zum Menschlischen Verhalten Unter Extremen
Lebensverhältnissen. [*Some Remarks on Human Behaviour in Extreme
Life Situations*]. Ärzt Prax (1960) 12:1–23.

10840   PAUL, H.A.
Die Psyche Des Hungernden Und Des Dystrophikers. [*The Psyche of
the Starving and Dystrophic Individual*]. In Extreme

Lebensverhältnisse Und Ihre Folgen. Bericht Über Den 4
Ärztekongress Für Pathologie, Therapie Und Begutachtung Der
Heimkehrerkrankheiten in Düsseldorf. Verband Der Heimkehrer,
1959, Band 8, 5– 127.

10850   PAUL, H.A.
Personality Study of Former Prisoners of War and Former Internees. In
Later Effects of Imprisonment and Deportation. International
Conference Organized by the World Veterans Federation. The Hague:
World Veterans Federation, 1961, 101– 106.

10860   PAUL, H.A.
*Problems in the Classification of Personality Disorders Following
Imprisonment.* In Later Effects of Imprisonment and Deportation.
International Conference Organized by the World Veterans
Federation. The Hague; World Veterans Federation, 1961, 107– 108.

10870   PAUL, H.A.; HERBERG, H.J.
Psychische Spätschäden Nach Verfolgungseinfluessen In Der
Kindheit Und Jugend. [*Psychological Sequelae after Persecution in
Childhood and Youth*]. In Paul, H. and H.J. Herberg (eds.), Psychische
Spätschäden Nach Politischer Verfolgung. Basel: S. Karger, 1963,
179– 206.

10880   PAUL, H.A.; HERBERG, H.J.
Psychische Spätschäden Nach Politischer Verfolgung. [*Psychological
Sequelae after Political Persecution*]. Basel: S. Karger, 1963. With
papers by von Baeyer, Doering, Haefner, Kluge, Mende, Bondy,
Herberg, Fitzek, Kisker, Lingens, Paul, Mengelberg, Venzlaff.

10890   PAUL, H.A.
Internationale Erfahrungen Mit Psychischen Spätschäden
[*International Experience with Psychological Sequelae*]. In Paul, H. and
H.J. Herberg (eds.), Psychische Spätschäden Nach Politischer
Verfolgung. Basel: S. Karger, 1963, 37– 84.

10900   PAUL, H.A.
Psychologische Untersuchungsergebnisse 15 Jahre Nach Der
Verfolgung. [*Results of Psychological Investigations 15 Years after the
Persecution*]. In Paul, H. and H.J. Herberg (eds.), Psychische
Spätschäden Nach Politischer Verfolgung. Basel: S. Karger, 1963,
207-243.

10910   PAUL, H.A.; HERBERG, H.J.
Psychische Spätschäden Nach Politischer Verfolgung. [*Psychic
Sequelae after Political Persecution*]. 2nd Ed. New York: Karger
Verlag, 1967. With papers of the same authors as in the first edition
and additional papers by Paul and Herberg.

10920   PAUL, H.A.
Neuere Studien Zum Thema. [*Newer Studies of the Problem*]. In Paul,
H. and H.J. Herberg (eds.), Psychische Spätschäden Nach Politischer
Verfolgung. Basel: S. Karger, 1967, 78– 138.

10930   PAUL, H.A.
Methodologische Probleme Bei Der Untersuchung Auf Psychische
Störungen Nach Gefangenschaft Und Verfolgung. [*Methodological
Problems in the Investigation of Psychological Disturbances after
Imprisonment and Persecution*]. In Herberg, H.J. (ed.), Die
Beurteilung Von Gesundheitsschäden Nach Gefangenschaft Und
Verfolgung. Internationalen Medizinisch-Juristischen Symposiums in
Köln, 1967. Herford: Nicholaische Verlagsbuchhandlung, 1967,
77–83.

10940   PAUL, H.A.
Vorzeitiger Verschleiss Nach Zwangsarbeit Unter Extremen
Verhältnissen. [*Premature Aging after Forced Labour under Extreme
Stress*]. Sonderdruck Aus "Arbeitswissenschaft." Mainz:
Krausskopf-Verlag, 1967, 4/5.

10950   PAUL, H.A.
Das Stressgeschehen In Verfolgung Und Gefangenschaft. [*The
Experience of Stress in Persecution and Imprisonment*]. In Herberg,
H.J. (ed.), Spätschäden Nach Extremebelastungen. II Internationalen
Medizinisch-Juristischen Konferenze in Düsseldorf, 1969. Herford:
Nicholaische Verlagsbuchhandlung, 1971, 21–28.

10960   PAUL-MENGELBERG, M.
Die Bedeutung Der Graphologischen Diagnostik Im Rahmen Der
Begutachtung Verfolgter. [*The Meaning of the Graphological Diagnosis
in the Frame of Evaluation of Persecutees*]. In Paul, H. and H.J.
Herberg (eds.), Psychische Spätschäden Nach Politischer Verfolgung.
Basel: S. Karger, 1963, 245–255.

10970   PAUL-MENGELBERG, M.
Schriftpsychologische Begutachtung Von Spätschäden Nach
Gefangenschaft Und Verfolgung. [*Psychological Evaluation of
Handwriting in Cases of Late Damage After Imprisonment and
Persecution*]. In Herberg, H.J. (ed.), Die Beurteilung Von
Gesundheitsschäden Nach Gefangenschaft Verfolgung.
Internationalen Medizinisch-Juristischen Symposiums in Köln, 1967.
Herford: Nicholaische Verlagsbuchhandlung, 1967, 84–92.

10980   PAUL-MENGELBERG, M.
Schreibmotorische Störungen Bei Ehemaligen Kriegsgefangenen Und
Verfolgten. [*Motor Disturbances in Writing in Former Prisoners of War
and Persecutees*]. In Herberg, H.J. (ed.), Spätschäden Nach
Extremebelastungen. II Internationalen Medizinisch-Juristischen
Konferenz in Düsseldorf (1969). Herford: Nicholaische
Verlagsbuchhandlung, 1971, 206–217.

10990   PAWELCZYNSKA, A.
[*Social Structural Changes and Prospects for Survival at the Auschwitz
Concentration Camp*]. Przeglad Lekarski (1973) 30(1):76–81.

11000   PAWLOWSKI, B.
[*The Concentration Camp Hospital at Wiener Neudorf*]. Przeglad
Lekarski (1974) 31(1):195–200.

11010 PAWLOWSKI, B.
[*Some Unknown Episodes at the Aflezn Concentration Camp*]. Przeglad Lekarski (1976) 33(1):188–194.

11020 PAWLOWSKI, B.
[*Arrival in Mauthausen*]. Przeglad Lekarski (1979) 36(1):156–159.

11030 PEDERSEN, S.
Psychopathological Reactions to Extreme Social Displacement (Refugee Neuroses). Psychoanal Rev (1949) 36:344–354.

11040 PELSER, H. E.
Latere gevolgen van verzet en vervolging: een psychosomatisch probleem. [*Later Sequelae of Resistance and Persecution: A Psychosomatic Problem*]. In Dane, J., Keerzijde van de bevrijding [*The Other Side of Liberation*]. Deventer, 1984.

11050 PERETZ, D.
Gormin Psihosomatiyim B'alveset. [*Psychosomatic Factors in Amenorrhea*]. Harefuah (1954) 46:189–192.

11055 PERL, G.
I Was a Doctor In Auschwitz. New York: Arno Books, 1979.

11060 PERL, J. L.; KAHN, M. W.
The Effects of Compensation on Psychiatric Disability. Soc Sci Med (1983) 17(7):439–443.

11070 PESKIN, H.
Observations on the First International Conference on Children of Holocaust Survivors. Fam Process (1981) 20:391–394.

11080 PFISTER-AMMENDE, M.
Psychologie Und Psychiatrie Der Internierung Und des Fluechtlingsdaseins. [*Psychology and Psychiatry of Internment and Refugees*]. In Gruhle, H. (ed.), Psychiatrie der Gegenwart, Vol. 3. Berlin: Springer, 1961.

11090 PHILLIPS, R. E.
Impact of Nazi Holocaust on Children of Survivors. Am J Psychother (1978) 32:370–378.

11100 PIEKARA, A. H.
Episodes from the So-Called Sonderaktion Krakau. Przeglad Lekarski (1979) 36(1):146–148.

11110 PIEKUT-WARSZAWSKA, E.
Reminiscences of a Nurse. In Auschwitz, In Hell They Preserved Human Dignity, Anthology, Vol. 2, Part 2. Warsaw: International Auschwitz Committee, 1971, 1–12.

11120 PIOREK, J.
The Gross-Rosen Camp. A Few Observations. Przeglad Lekarski (1976) 33(1):184–188.

11130   PODIETZ, L.
        The Holocaust Revisited in the Next Generation. Analysis: Jewish
        Institute for Policy Studies Bull (1975) 1– 5.

11140   PODIETZ, L.; ZWERLING, I.; FICHER, I.; BELMONT, H.;
        EISENSTEIN, T.; SHAPIRO, M.; LEVICK, M.
        Engagement in Families of Holocaust Survivors. J Mar Fam Ther
        (1984) 10:43– 51.

11150   PODLAHA, J.; ZEMAN, F.
        Dauerfolgen Des Hungers in Den Konzentrationslagern. [*Longterm
        Sequels of Famine in the Concentration Camps*]. In Ätio-Pathogenese
        Und Therapie Der Erschoepfung Und Vorzeitigen Vergreisung. IV
        Internationaler Medizinischer Kongress Der F.I.R. Bucharest: Verlag
        Der F.I.R., 1964, 114– 118.

11160   PODLAHA, J.; ZEMAN, F.
        Das Hungerödem Und Sein Einfluss Auf Die Arterien Der Unteren
        Extremitäten. [*The Edema of Famine and its Influence on the Arteries
        of the Lower Extremities*]. In Die Behandlung Der Asthenie Und Der
        Vorzeitigen Vergreisung Bei Ehemaligen Widerstanskämpfern Und
        KZ Häftlingen. III Internationale Medizinisch Konferenz. Liège:
        Verlag Der F.I.R., 1964, 114– 118.

11170   POLAK, B. S.
        De rol van de huisarts bij de signalering en behandeling van
        psychosomatische klachten van oorlogsgetroffenen. [*The Role of the
        General Practitioner in the Recognition and Treatment of
        Psychosomatic Complaints of War Victims*]. In Dane, J., Keerzijde van
        de Bevrijding. [*The Other Side of Liberation*]. Deventer, 1984,
        190– 203.

11180   POLAK, G.
        "Massive Social Trauma," enige opmerkingen over de situatie van
        vervolgingsslachtoffers. [*"Massive Social Trauma," Some Remarks on
        the Situation of Victims of Persecution*]. Jerusalem, 1977. Manuscript.

11190   POLIEZER, M.
        Über Störungen Der Schildruesenfunktion Und Deren Beeinflussung
        Bei Den Opfern Des Faschismus. [*Disturbances of the Thyroid
        Function in Victims of Fascism*]. In Die Behandlung Der Asthenie
        Und Der Vorzeitigen Vergreisung Bei Ehemaligen
        Widerstanskämpfern Und KZ Häftlingen. III Internationale
        Medizinische Konferenz. Liège: Verlag Der F.I.R., 1961, 119– 125.

11200   POLTAWSKA, W. Z.
        Badania Nad "Dziecmi Oswiecimskimi" (Uwagi Ogolne). [*From the
        Research on the So-Called "Auschwitz-Children" General
        Considerations*]. In Piaty Zeszyt Poswiecony Zagadnieniom Lekarskim
        Okresu Hitlerowskiej Okupacji. Przeglad Lekarski (1965) 21(1):21– 24.

11210   POLTAWSKA, W.; JAKUBIK, A.; SARNECKI, J.; GATARSKI, J.
        Wyniki Badan Psychiatrycznych Osob Urodzonych Lub Wiezionych
        W Cziecinstwie W Hitlerowskich Obozach Koncentracyjanych.

[*Results of the Psychiatric Studies of Persons Either Born or Imprisoned in Childhood in Hitlerian Concentration Camps*]. Przeglad Lekarski (1966) 23:21–36.

11220 POLTAWSKA, W.
On Examinations of "Auschwitz Children." In Auschwitz, In Hell They Preserved Human Dignity, Anthology, Vol. 2, Part 2. Warsaw: International Auschwitz Committee, 1971, 21–36.

11230 POLTAWSKA, W.
"Guinea Pigs" in the Ravensbruck Concentration Camp. In Auschwitz, Inhuman Medicine, Anthology, Vol. 1, Part 2. Warsaw: International Auschwitz Committee, 1971, 131–162.

11240 POLTAWSKA, W.
Anfälle Von Paroxismaler Hypermnesie Bei Ehemaligen Häftlingen, Beobachtet Nach 30 Jahren. [*States of Paroxysmal Hypermnesia in Ex-Prisoners Observed 30 Years Later*]. VI Internationaler Medizinischer Kongress Der F.I.R., Prague, 1976, 85–94.

11250 POLTAWSKA, W.
Anfälle Von Paroxismaler Hypermnesie (auf Grund von Untersuchungen sog. ."Auschwitzkinder." [*Attacks of Paroxysmal Hypermnesia (Based on the Research in So-Called "Auschwitz Children"*]. Presented at VI Internationaler Medizinischer Kongress Der F.I.R. Prague, 30 November–2 December 1976.

11260 POLTAWSKA, W.
Stany Hipermnezji Napadowej U Bylych Wiezniow Obserwowane Po 30 Latach [*States of Paroxysmal Hypermnesia in Ex-Prisoners, Observed after 30 Years*]. Przeglad Lekarski (1978) 35:20–24.

11270 POMERANTZ, B.
Children of Survivors of The Holocaust: Perceptions of Their Need for Social Work and Community Services. MSW Thesis, University of Southern California, 1977.

11280 POMERANTZ, B.
Group Work with Children of Holocaust Survivors. Proceedings of the North American Symposium on Family Practice. New York: Family Service Association of America (1980) 194–203.

11290 POPEK, W.
W Rewirze Obozu W Gross-Rosen. [*In the Sick Bay of the Concentration Camp Gross-Rosen*]. Przeglad Lekarski (1978) 35:171–172.

11300 POPPER, L.
Ärztliche Erfahrungen Bei Untersuchungen Nach Dem Österreichischen Opferfürsorgegesetz. [*Medical Experience in Investigations According to the Austrian Law of Compensation*]. In Michel, M. (ed.), Gesundheitsschäden Durch Verfolgung Und Gefangenschaft Und Ihre Spätfolgen. Frankfurt Am Main: Roederberg Verlag, 1955, 281–287.

11310   PORTER, J. N.
Social Psychological Aspects of the Holocaust. In B. L. Sherwin and
G. S. Ament (eds.), Encountering the Holocaust. Chicago: Impact
Press, 1979, 189–222.

11320   PORTER, J. N.
*Is There a Survivor Syndrome? Psychological and Socio-Political
Implications.* J Psychol Judaism (1981) 6(1):33–52.

11330   POZNANIAK, W.
*The Stress Mechanism of the Desocialization of the Personality of a
Concentration Camp Prisoner: Introductory Psychological Analysis.*
Przeglad Psychologiczny (1972) 15(2):29–44.

11340   PRAAG, Van J. P.
*Background, Problems and Possibilities of Treatment in Cases of
Extreme Stress.* In Israel-Netherlands Symposium on the Impact of
Persecution, Jerusalem, 1977. The Netherlands: Rijswijk, 1979, 9–17.

11350   PRINCE, R. M.
*Psychohistorial Themes in the Lives of Young Adult Children of
Concentration Camp Survivors.* Ph.D. diss., Columbia University, 1975.
Page 1453 in Vol 36/03-B of Dissertation Abstracts International.
Order No.: AAD75-18431.

11360   PRINCE, R. M.
*A Case Study of a Psychohistorical Figure: The Influence of the
Holocaust on Identity.* J Contemp Psychother (1980) 11(1):44–60.

11370   PRZYCHODZKI, M.
[*Physicians from the Great Poland Region during the Nazi
Occupation—A Martyrdom*]. Przeglad Lekarski (1978) 35(1):116–131.

11380   QUAYTMAIN, W.
(Ed.). *Holocaust Survivors: Psychological and Social Sequelae.* Special
Issue of Journal of Contemporary Psychotherapy (1980) 2(1).

11390   RABKIN, L. Y.
*Countertransference in the Extreme Situation: The Family Therapy of
Survivor Families.* In Wolberg, L. R. and M. L. Aronson (eds.), Group
Therapy: An Overview. New York: Stratton Intercontinental, 1975.

11400   RABKIN, L. Y.; KRELL, R.
The Transmission of Effects in Holocaust Families. Presented at
International Scholars Symposium on Western Society after the
Holocaust, Seattle, Washington, November 1978. Manuscript.

11410   RADIL-WEISS, T.
*Men In Extreme Conditions: Some Medical and Psychological Aspects
of the Auschwitz Concentration Camp.* Psychiat (1983) 46:259–269.

11420   RAKOFF, V.
Long Term Effects of the Concentration Camp Experience. Viewpoint.
Labour Zionist Movement of Canada (1966) 1:17–21.

11430 RAKOFF, V.; SIGAL, J.J.; EPSTEIN, N.B.
Children and Families of Concentration Camp Survivors. Can Ment Health (1966) 24–26.

11440 RAPPAPORT, E.A.
Beyond Traumatic Neurosis: A Psychoanalytic Study of Late Reactions to Concentration Camp Trauma. Int J Psychoanal (1968) 49:719–731.

11450 RAPPAPORT, E.A.
Survivor Guilt. Midstream (1971) 27:41–47.

11460 RAVEAU, F.A.
Neuropsychiatric Data on the State of Health of Former Deportees Fifteen Years after Their Liberation. In Experts Meeting on the Effects of Imprisonment and Deportation, Oslo, 1960. Paris: World Veterans Federation, 1960, 79–88.

11470 RAVEAU, F.A.
Neuropsychiatric Study of Former Deportees. General Conclusions. In Later Effects of Imprisonment and Deportation. International Conference Organized by the World Veterans Federation, 1961, 109–110.

11480 RAVESTEIJN, Van, L.
De arts geconfronteerd met lijders aan het KZ-Syndroome. [*The Physician Confronted with Patients Suffering from the Concentration Camp Syndrome*]. Neederl Tijdschr Geneesk (1976) 120:316–318.

11490 RAVESTEIJN, Van, L.
Gelaagdheid van herinneringen [*The Characteristics of Memories*]. Tijdschr Psychother (1976) 5:195–205.

11500 RAVESTEIJN, Van, L.
De Traumatische Droom. [*The Traumatic Dream*]. Tijdschr Psychother (1976) 2:1–8.

11510 RAVESTEIJN, Van, L.
Gelaagdheid van emoties, het "onzichtbare" schaamtegevoel en het KZ-Syndroome. [*The Characteristics of Emotions, the Invisible Feelings of Shame in the Concentration Camp Syndrome*]. Tijdschr Psychother (1978) 4:175–185.

11520 REICH, S.
Ohrenkrankheitsfolgen Einige Aspekte Der Durch Verletzung Entstandenen Taubheit Bei Den Ehemaligen Deportierten. [*Sequels of Ear Diseases. Some Aspects of Deafness Caused by Trauma in Ex-Deportees*]. In Michel, M. (ed.), Gesundheitsschäden Durch Verfolgung Und Gefangenschaft Und Ihre Spätfolgen. Frankfurt Am Main: Röderberg Verlag, 1955, 216–224. Also in Fichez, L.F., Andere Spätfolgen. Austria: Verlag Der F.I.R., 1959, 173–183.

11530 REWERTS, G.
Die Akuten Neurologischen Syndrome Bein Hungernden. [*The Acute Neurological Syndromes in the Starving Individual*]. In Extreme

Lebensverhältnisse Und Ihre Folkgen. Bericht Über Den 4
Ärztekongress Für Pathologie, Therapie Und Begutachtung Der
Heimkehrerkrankheiten in Düsseldorf, 1959. Verband Der
Heimkehrer, 1959, Band 8 128–172.

11540   RICH, M. S.
*Children of Holocaust Survivors. A Concurrent Validity Study of a
Survivor Family Typology.* Ph.D. diss., California School of
Professional Psychology, Berkeley. Page 1626 in Vol 43/05-B of
Dissertation Abstracts International. Order No: AAD82-23533.

11550   RICHARTZ, M.
Zur Frage Der Wesentlichen Mitverursachung Schizophrener
Psychosen Durch Verfolgungsbedingte Extremebelastungen. [*The
Question of Contribution to Schizophrenia Psychoses by Extreme Stress
Caused by Persecution*]. VI Internationaler Medizinischer Kongress
Der F.I.R., Prague, 1976.

11560   RICHET, C.; GILBERT-DREYFUSS, H.; UZAN, H.; FICHEZ, L. F.
Die Folgeerscheinungen Des Physiologischen Elendszustandes. [*The
Sequelae of Physiological Misery*]. In Michel, M. (ed.),
Gesundheitsschaeder Durch Verfolgung Und Gefangenschaft Und Ihre
Spätfolgen. Frankfurt Am Main: Röderberg Verlag, 1955, 73–81.

11570   RICHET, C.; PARISOT; DESOILLE, H.; ELLENBOGEN, R.; FICHEZ,
L. F.; GALLET; GILBERT-DREYFUSS, H.; MANS, A.; SEGELLE;
UZAN.
Les Sequelles de la Misère chez l'Adulte. [*The Effects of Misery in
Adults*]. Bull Acad Nat Méd (1955) 139:245–250.

11580   RICHET, C.; MANS, A.
Pathologie de la Déportation. [*The Pathology of Deportation*]. [N.P.]:
A.D.I.F. Des Alpes-Maritimes et de la Principalité de Monaco, 1958.

11590   RICHET, C.; MANS, A.
Delayed Cardiovascular Aftereffects among Former Deportees. In
Experts Meeting on the Later Effects of Imprisonment and
Deportation. Oslo, 1960. Paris: World Veterans Federation, 1960,
13–19.

11600   RICHET, C.
Introduction. In Experts Meeting on the Later Effects of
Imprisonment and Deportation, Oslo, 1960. Paris: World Veterans
Federation, 1960, 7–11.

11610   RICHET, C.
Introduction. In Later Effects of Imprisonment and Deportation.
International Conference Organized by the World Veterans
Federation. The Hague: World Veterans Federation, 1961, 23–26.

11620   RICHMAN, L.
From the Family Album. In Steinitz, L. (ed.), Living after the
Holocaust: Reflections by the Post-War Generation. New York: Bloch,
1975, 131–135.

11630   RIECK, M.; EITINGER, L.
A Critical Review of the Literature Concerning the Sequels

of the Holocaust in Survivors. Paper presented at the World Congress on Behavior Therapy, Jerusalem, 13– 17 July 1980. Manuscript.

11640 RIECK, M.; EITINGER, L.
Psychological Investigations of Holocaust Survivors' Offspring. University of Haifa, Ray D. Wolfe Centre for Study of Psychological Stress. Manuscript.

11650 RIIS, P.
The Many Faces of Inhumanity—and the Few Faces of Its Psychic and Somatic Sequelae. Dan Med Bull (1980) 27(5):213– 214.

11660 ROBINSON, S.; AHARONSON, R.
Manganonei Hagfana Vehimidedut Sh'Azru Behistaglut Etsel Nitsolei Hasho'ah. [*Defensive and Coping Mechanisms That Helped in the Adaptation of Survivors*]. Israel's 3rd Meeting of the Psychiatric Association, 1974. Manuscript.

11670 ROBINSON, S.
Holocaust Survivors' Attitudes toward Death. In De Vries, A. and A. Carmi (eds.), The Dying Human. Ramat-Gan: Turtledove Publishing, 1979, 1– 8.

11680 ROBINSON, S.
Late Effects of Persecution in Persons Who As Children or Young Adolescents Survived Nazi Occupation in Europe. Isr Ann Psychiat Rel Disc (1979) 17(3):209– 214.

11690 ROBINSON, S.; WINNIK, H. Z.
Second Generation of the Holocaust. Holocaust Survivors' Communication of Experience to Their Children, and Its Effects. Isr J Psychiat Rel Sci (1981) 18:99– 107.

11700 ROBINSON, S.; HEMMENDINGER, J.
Psychosocial Adjustment 30 Years Later of People Who Were in Nazi Concentration Camps as Children. In Milgram, N. (ed.), Stress and Anxiety. Washington: Hemisphere, 1982, 397– 399.

11710 RODEN, R.G.; RODEN, M.M.
Children of Holocaust Survivors. Adolesc Psychiat (1982) 10:66– 72.

11720 RODEN, R.G.
Suicide and Holocaust Survivors. Isr J Psychiat Rel Sci (1982) 19(2):129– 135.

11730 ROGAN, B.
Criteria to be Considered for the Evaluation of Disability. In Experts Meeting on the Later Effects of Imprisonment and Deportation. Oslo, 1960. Paris: World Veterans Federation, 1960, 143– 148.

11740 ROGAN, B.
Introduction. In Experts Meeting on the Later Effects of Imprisonment and Deportation, Oslo, 1960. Paris: World Veterans Federation, 1960, 143– 148.

11750 ROGAN, B.
Short Survey of an Investigation Carried Out in Norway on Medical

Problems of Camp Survivors. In Experts Meeting on the Later Effects of Imprisonment and Deportation, Oslo, 1960. Paris: World Veterans Federation, 1960, 99–106.

11760   ROGAN, B.
Social and Vocational Problems of Ex-Concentration Camp Prisoners. In Later Effects of Imprisonment and Deportation, International Conference Organized by the World Veterans Federation. The Hague: World Veterans Federation, 1961, 162–166.

11770   ROGAN, B.
Sosiale Og Yrkesmessige Forhold Hos Tidligere Konsentrasjonsleirfanger. [*Social and Professional Problems of Ex-Concentration Camp Prisoners*]. Tidsskr Norske Laegeforening (1961) 81:812–815.

11780   ROMBERG, P.
Understanding and Helping the Survivors of the Nazi Concentration Camps. 1974. Manuscript.

11790   ROSE, H.K.
Zur Frage Der Wesentlichen Mitverursachung Schizophrener Psychosen Durch Verfolgungsbedingte Extremebelastungen. [*The Problem of Causal Relationship Between Schizophrenic Psychoses and Extreme Stress Caused by Persecution*]. VI Internationaler Medizinischer Kongress Der F.I.R., Prague, 1976.

11800   ROSE, S.L.
Adaptive Behavior and Coping among Children of Holocaust Survivors: Controlled Comparative Investigation. Ph.D. diss., Ohio University, 1983. Page 2905 in Vol 44/09-B of Dissertation Abstracts International. Order No AAD83-29150.

11810   ROSENBERGER, L.
Children of Survivors. In Anthony, E.J. and C. Koupernik (eds.), The Child in His Family: The Impact of Disease and Death. New York: Wiley, 1973, 375–377.

11820   ROSENBLOOM, M.
Implications of the Holocaust for Social Work. Soc Casework (1983) 64(4):205–213.

11830   ROSENKOTTER, L.
[*Shadow of History upon Psychoanalytic Therapy*]. Psyche (1979) 33(11):1024–1038.

11840   ROSENMAN, S.
Compassion Versus Contempt toward Holocaust Victims: Difficulties in Attaining an Adaptive Identity in an Annihilative World. Isr J Psychiat Rel Sci (1982) 19:39–73.

11850   ROSENMAN, S.
The Psychoanalytic Writer on the Holocaust and Bettelheim. Am J Soc Psychiat (1984) 4(2):62–71.

11860 ROSENTHAL, P.A.; ROSENTHAL, S.
Holocaust Effect in the Third Generation: Child of Another Time. Am J
Psychother (1980) 34(4):572–580.

11870 ROTENBERG, L.A.
A Child Survivor/Psychiatrist's Personal Adaptation. Presented at the
APA Symposium on Child Survivors of the Holocaust—40 Years
Later. Los Angeles, 1984. J Amer Acad Child Psychiat. July, 1985.

11880 ROZEN, R.
Depression and Anxiety in Holocaust Survivors. Ph.D. diss., California
School of Professional Psychology, Los Angeles, 1983. Page 3540 in
Vol 44/11-B of Dissertation Abstracts International. Order No:
AAD84-00528.

11890 RUBENSTEIN, I.
*Multi-generational Occurrence of Survivor Syndrome Symptoms in the
Families of Holocaust Survivors.* Ph.D. diss., California School of
Professional Psychology, Fresno, 1981. Page 4209 in Vol 42/10-B of
Dissertation Abstracts International. Order No AAD82-07545.

11900 RUDOWSKI, W.
[*The Last Illness of General Stefan Grot-Rowecki (1895–1944)*]. Arch
Hist Med (Wars) (1983) 46(4):475–480.

11910 RÜMKE, H.C.
Late Werkingen Van Psychotraumata. [*Late Consequences of Psychic
Trauma*]. Ned Tijdschr Geneesk (1951) 95:2928–2937.

11920 RUSINEK, K.
[*Ceremony at Mauthausen in Honour of Interned Physicians. Dr.
Wladyslaw Czaplinski*]. Przeglad Lekarski (1979) 36(1):124–131.

11930 RUSSELL, A.
*Late Psychosocial Consequences in Concentration Camp Survivors
Families.* Am J Orthopsychiat (1974) 44(4):611–619.

11940 RUSSELL, A.
*Late Effects—Influence on the Children of the Concentration Camp
Survivors.* In Dimsdale, J.E. (ed.), Survivors, Victims and
Perpetrators. Washington: Hemisphere, 1980, 175–203.

11950 RUSSELL, A.
*Late Psychosocial Consequences of the Holocaust Experience on
Survivor Families: The Second Generation.* Int J Fam Psychiat (1982)
3:375–402.

11960 RUSSELL, A.
*Family/Marital Therapy with Second Generation Holocaust Survivor
Families, Questions and Answers.* In Gurman, A. (ed.), The Practice of
Family Therapy, Vol. 2. New York: Brunner Mazel, 1982, 233–237.

11970 RUSSELL, A.
A Comparison of Adaptive and Coping Abilities in Non-Clinical Second

Generation Survivor Families and Non-Holocaust North American Controls. 1984. Manuscript.

11980   RUSTIN, S.L.; LIPSIG, F.S.
Psychotherapy with the Adolescent Children of Concentration Camp Survivors. J Contemp Psychother (1972) 4(2):87–94.

11990   RUSTIN, S.L.
Offspring of Survivors Compared with Jewish Adolescents. (1979) 93–95. Manuscript.

12000   RUSTIN, S.L.
Guilt, Hostility and Jewish Identification Among a Self-Selected Sample of Adolescent Children of Jewish Concentration Camp Survivors: A Descriptive Study. Ph.D. diss., City University of New York, 1971. Page 1859 in Vol 32/03-B of Dissertation Abstracts International. Order No: AAD71-24810.

12010   RUSTIN, S.L.
The Legacy is Loss. J Contemp Psychother (1980) 11(1):32–43.

12020   RYN, Z.; KLODZINSKI, S.
[Pathology of Sport at the Auschwitz-Birkenau Concentration Camp]. Przeglad Lekarski (1974) 31(1):46–58.

12030   RYN, Z.; KLODZINSKI, S.
The Problem of Suicides in Nazi Concentration Camps. VI Internationaler Medizinischer Kongress Der F.I.R., Prague, 1976.

12040   RYN, Z.; KLODZINSKI, S.
[Suicides in Nazi Concentration Camps]. Przeglad Lekarski (1976) 33(1):25–46.

12050   RYN, Z.; KLODZINSKI, S.
[Hunger in the Concentration Camp]. Przeglad Lekarski (1984) 41(1):21–37.

12060   RYN, Z.
Z Badan Nad Zachorowalnoscia Smieretloscia Bylych Wiezniow Obozow Koncentracyjnych. [The Research in Mortality and Morbidity of Ex-Concentration Camp Survivors]. Przeglad Lekarski (1977) 34(1):1–15.

12070   RYN, Z.
Z Psychologii I Psychopatologii Obozow Koncentracyjnych I Jenieckich. Przeglad Pismiennictwa Zachodniegoi. [On the Psychology and Psychopathology of the Concentration Camps. A Survey of the Western Literature]. Przeglad Lekarski (1978) 35:231–237.

12080   RYN, Z.
[Antoni Kepinski at the Miranda de Ebro Concentration Camp]. Przeglad Lekarski (1978) 35(1):95–115.

12090   RYN, Z.
[A Psychiatrist's Remarks on the So-Called Concentration Camp Syndrome]. Przeglad Lekarski (1981) 38(10):26–29.

12100 RYN, Z.
The Evolution of Mental Disturbances in the Concentration Camp Syndrome. In Cah d'inf méd soc jurid (1983) 19:209–223.

12110 RYN, Z.
Death and Dying in the Concentration Camp. Am J Soc Psychiat (1983) 3(3):32–38.

12120 SACHS, L.J.; TITIEVSKY, J.
On Identification with the Aggressor: A Clinical Note. Isr Ann Psychiat All Disc (1967) 5:181–184.

12130 SALLER, K.
Anlagebedingt. [*"Caused by Disposition"*]. Wiedergutmachungs-Beilage (1960) (6).

12140 SALLER, K.
Gutachten Über Vorzeitiges Entpflichtung Verfolgter Des Naziregimes. [*Expert Statement on Premature Retirement of Nazi Persecutees*]. In Ätio-Pathogenese Und Therapie Der Erschöpfung Und Vorzeitigen Vergreisung. IV Internationaler Medizinischer Kongress Der F.I.R. Bucharest: Verlag Der F.I.R., 1964, 568–572.

12150 SALLER, K.
Erb Und Umwelteinfluesse Bei "Anlageleiden." [*The Influence of Genetics and Environment in Diseases "Caused by" Disposition*]. In Herberg, H.J. (ed.), Spätschäden Nach Extremebelastungen. II Internationalen Medizinisch-Juristischen Konferenz in Düsseldorf, 1969. Herford: Nicholaische Verlagsbuchhandlung, 1971, 13–20.

12160 SALZBERGER,
Problems of Providing Care for Survivors of the Second World-War. In Israel-Netherlands Symposium on the Impact of Persecution, Jerusalem, 1977. The Netherlands: Rijswijk, 1979, 74–75.

12170 SANDLER, J.
Trauma, Strain and Development. In S.S. Furst (ed.), Psychic Trauma. New York: Basic Books, 1967.

12180 SARNECKI, J.
Konflikty Emocjonalne Osob Urodzonych Lub Wieznionych W Dziecinstwie W Hitlerowskich Obozach Koncentracyjnych. [*Emotional Conflicts in Persons Born in Hitlerian Concentration Camps or Arrested in Their Earliest Childhood*]. Przeglad Lekarski (1966) 23:39–46.

12190 SARNECKI, J.
Emotional Conflicts of People Born in Nazi Concentration Camps or Imprisoned There During Their Childhood. In Auschwitz, Anthology, Vol. 2, Part 3. Warsaw: International Auschwitz Committee, 1971, 143–189.

12200 SAVRAN, B.; FOGELMAN, E.
Therapeutic Groups for Children of Holocaust Survivors. Int J Group Psychother (1979) 29:211–215.

12210   SCHACHTER, M.
Le Syndrome Neuro-Psychiatrique Séquellaire des Anciens Deportés
et Persecutés Non-Deportes à la Lumière du Test de Rorschach. [Late
Neuro-Psychiatric Problems in Ex-Deportees and Non-Deported
Persecutees as Demonstrated in the Rorschach Test.]. Giornale Psichiat
Neuropatol (1965) 93:153– 186.

12220   SCHAPPES, M.
Holocaust and Resistance. A Response on Receiving the Holocaust
Memorial Award of the New York Society of Clinical Psychologists.
(A Special Issue). J Contemp Psychother (1980) 11(1):61– 69.

12230   SCHATZKER, C.
The Teaching of the Holocaust—Dilemmas and Considerations. In
Israel-Netherlands Symposium on the Impact of Persecution. 2,
Dalfsen, Amsterdam, 14– 18 April 1980. The Netherlands: Rijswijk,
1981, 79– 84.

12240   SCHENCK, E.G.
Alterung Und Anlage. [Aging and Disposition]. In Extreme
Lebensverhältnisse Und Irhe Folgen. Bericht Über Den 4
Ärztekongress Für Pathologie, Therapie Und Begutachtung Der
Heimkehrerkrankheiten in Düsseldorf (1959), Band 8, 16– 33.

12250   SCHENCK, E.G.; NATHUSIUS, Von, W.
Extreme Lebensverhältnisse Und Ihre Folgen. [Extreme Life
Situations and Their Sequelae]. Verbandes Der Heimkehrer, 1961,
Band 5. Papers by: Paul, Rewerts, Muehlbaecher.

12260   SCHENCK, E.G.; SCHEID, G.
Die Folgen Extremer Lebensverhältnisse Bei Gefangener Und
Internierten Und Ihre Beurteilung. [The Sequelae of Extreme Life
Situations in Prisoners and Internees, and Their Evaluation]. Internist
(1965) 6:276– 284.

12270   SCHENCK, E.G.
[Premature Aging Resulting from Exogenous Factors and Endogenous
Predisposition]. Ther Ggw (1977) 116(3):446– 450, 455– 470.

12280   SCHIFFER, I.
The Trauma of Time. Analysis of a Concentration Camp Survivor. New
York: International Universities Press, 1978.

12290   SCHMALE, Jr., A.H.
Psychic Trauma during Bereavement. In Krystal, H. and G. Niederland
(eds.), Massive Traumatization. Boston: Little, Brown, (1970)
147– 168.

12300   SCHMIDT, D.
Probleme Der Zweiten Generation Aus Internistischer Sicht.
[Problems of the Second Generation as Seen in Internal Medicine]. VI
Internationaler Medizinischer Kongress Der F.I.R., Prague, 1976,
61– 63.

12310   SCHMIDT, S.
[Memoirs From Barracks 46 in Sachsenhausen]. Przeglad Lekarski
(1977) 34(1):191– 193.

12320   SCHNEIDER, G.
        Survival and Guilt Feelings of Jewish Concentration Camp Victims.
        Jewish Soc St (1975) 37:74–83.

12330   SCHNEIDER, S.
        Attitudes toward Death in Adolescent Offspring of Holocaust Survivors.
        Adolescence (1978) 13:575–584.

12340   SCHNEIDER, S.
        A Proposal for Treating Adolescent Offspring of Holocaust Survivors. J
        Psychol Judaism (1981) 6:68–76.

12350   SCHROEDER, A.
        Betrieft Kriegskörperschäden. [*On Body Damage due to War*]. VI
        Internationaler Medizinischer Kongress Der F.I.R., Prague, 1976.

12360   SCHWABER, E.
        *Reflections in Response to "A Psychoanalytic Overview on Children of
        Survivors," by Judith S. Kestenberg.* Symposium on The Psychology of
        the Jewish Experience: The Holocaust: Psychological Effects on
        Survivors and Their Children. Brandeis University, 21 May 1978.
        Manuscript.

12370   SCHWANN-PAWLOWSKA, J.
        Wstepne Wyniki Badan Lekarskich Bylych Wiezniow Hitlerowskich
        Obozow Koncentracyjnych. [*Preliminary Results of a Medical
        Investigation of Ex-Concentration Camp Prisoners*]. Przeglad Lekarski
        (1967) 24:98–101.

12380   SCHWANN-PAWLOWSKA, J.
        The Szczecin Environment. In Auschwitz, Anthology, Vol. 3, Part 1.
        Warsaw: International Auschwitz Committee, 1971, 171–179.

12385   SCHWARBERG, G.
        The Murders at Bullenhuser Damm: The SS Doctor and the Children.
        (Translation by E. B. Rosenfeld and A. H. Rosenfeld). Bloomington:
        Indiana University Press, 1984.

12390   SEDAN J.
        [*Sequelae of Oculary Lesions in Deportees to the Concentration Camps
        of 1943–1944*]. Bull Soc Optamol Fr (1965) 9:728–733.

12400   SEGAL, E.
        Tatspiyot R'fuiyot-psikholoqiyot bitkufat Hashoa.
        [*Medical-Psychological Observations in the Time of Disaster*]. Higena
        Ruhanit (1947/48) 5:103–108.

12410   SEGAL, J.
        *Long-Term Psychological and Physical Effects of the POW Experience: A
        Review of the Literature.* 1973. Report No 74-2, U. S. Naval Health
        Research Center, San Diego.

12420   SEGAL, J.; HUNTER, E. J.; SEGAL, Z.
        *Universal Consequences of Captivity: Stress Reactions among Divergent
        Populations of Prisoners of War and Their Families.* Int Soc Sci J
        (1976) 28:593–606.

12430   SEGALL, A.
Spätreaktion Auf Konzentrationslagererlebnisse. [*Late Reaction to Experiences of the Concentration Camps*]. Psyche (1971) 28:221–230.

12440   SEGELLE, P.; ELLENBOGAN, R.
Fréquence et Gravité des Différents Affections et Infirmités Recontrées chez les Survivants des Camps de Concentration. [*The Frequency and Seriousness of Different Problems and Diseases in the Survivors of Concentration Camps*]. Copenhagen: Congresverslag, 1954.

12450   SEGEV, T.
The Commanders of the Nazi Concentration Camps. Ph.D. diss., Boston University Graduate School, 1977. University Microfilms, Ann Arbor, Michigan, 77–21, 618.

12460   SEHN, J.
Some of the Legal Aspects of the So-Called Experiments Carried Out by SS Physicians in Concentration Camps. In Auschwitz, Inhuman Medicine, Anthology, Vol. 1, Part 1. Warsaw: International Auschwitz Committee, 1970, 43–84.

12470   SEHN, J.
The Case of the Auschwitz SS Physician, J. P. Kremer. In Auschwitz, Inhuman Medicine, Anthology, Vol. 1, Part 1. Warsaw: International Auschwitz Committee, 1970, 206–258.

12480   SEIDEL, K.
Über Psychische Spätschäden Bei Ehemaligen KZ-Häftlingen. [*Late Psychic Sequelae in Ex-Concentration Camp Prisoners*]. VI Internationaler Medizinischer Kongress Der F.I.R., Prague, 1976.

12490   SEIFERT, W.
[*The Holocaust and the Cultural Psychology of Sigmund Freud*]. Klin Psychol Psychother (1980) 28(4):292–301.

12500   SELAVAN, I. C.
Behavior Disorders of Jews: A Review of the Literature. J Psychol Judaism (1979) 4(2):117–124.

12510   SHAFIR, A.; HIRSCH, M.; SHEPPS, S.; RATZON, H.; SHALIT, B.; BRULL, F.
Hahaashpah Hanafshit Hameucheret Shel Chavajot Hashoa Kefi Shemishtdakefet Bemaarechet Mivchanin Psychodiagnostiim. [*The Delayed Mental Influence of the Holocaust Experience as Projected in a Psychodiagnostic Battery*]. Mental Health Clinic, Tel Aviv University Medical School, Kupat Holim, Tel Aviv. Manuscript.

12520   SHAMPO, M. A.; KYLE, R. A.
Henryk Goldszmit (1879–1942). J Am Med Ass (1975) 234(10):1042.

12530   SHANON, J.
Stress and Conflict as Criteria for the Classification of Psychosomatic Skin Disorders. Archives Belges de Dermatologie et de Syphiligraphie (1969) 25:429–437.

12540   SHANON, J.
Delayed Psychosomatic Skin Disorders in Survivors of Concentration Camps. Brit J Dermatology (1970) 83:536–542.

12550   SHANON, J.
Psychosomatic Skin Disorders in Survivors of Nazi Concentration Camps. Psychosomatics (1970) 2:95–98.

12560   SHANON, J.
Psychogenic Pruritus in Concentration Camp Survivors. (Delayed Psychosomatic Skin Disorders). Dynamic Psychiatry (1979) 56:232–241.

12570   SHANON, J.
The Subconscious Motivation for the Appearance of Psychosomatic Skin Disorders in Concentration Camp Survivors and Their Rehabilitation. Psychosomatics (1962) 3:178–182.

12580   SHAPIRO, M. H.
Psychophysiological Sequelae of Holocaust Trauma in a Jewish Child. Am J Psychoanal (1980) XL:53–66.

12600   SHEPS, J.
Ätio-Pathogenese Und Therapie Der Erschöpfung Und Vorzeitigen Vergreisung. [*The Aetiology, Pathogenesis, and Therapy of Exhaustion and Premature Aging*]. In Ätio-Pathogenese Und Therapie Der Erschöpfung Und Vorzeitigen Vergreisung. IV Internationaler Medizinischer Kongress Der F.I.R. Bucharest: Verlag Der F.I.R., 1964, 97–101.

12610   SHEPS, J.
Medical Observations on Proposed Changes in the Federal Compensation Law Relative to Damage to Health Caused by National Socialist Persecution. Manuscript. U. of Haifa (undated).

12620   SHEPS, J.
Organische Hirnschäden Bei Überlebenden Aus Konzentrationslagern in Den Vereinigten Staaten-Langfristige Reaktion Auf Extreme Unweltbelastungen. [*Organic Brain Damages in Concentration Camp Survivors in USA—Late Sequelae of Extreme Distress*]. In Herberg, H. J. (ed.), Spätschäden Nach Extremebelastungen. II Internationalen Medizinisch-Juristischen Konferenz in Düsseldorf, 1969. Herford: Nicholaische Verlagsbuchhandlung, 1971, 165–175.

12630   SHIBOLET, R.
Kiezen of delen, een visie over de ontwikkeling van de na-oorlogse joodse generatie in Nederland. [*Taking or Leaving it—A Vision on the Development of the Post-War Jewish Generation in the Netherlands*]. Doctoral thesis, University of Amsterdam, 1982.

12640   SHIRYON, S.
The Second Generation Leaves Home: The Function of the Sibling Subgroup in the Separation-Individuation Process of the Survivor Family. Ph.D. diss., The Wright Institute, 1982. Page 3376 in Vol

43/10-B of Dissertation Abstracts International. Order No:
AAD83-05602.

12650   SHUVAL, J. T.
*Some Persistent Effects of Trauma: Five Years after the Nazi
Concentration Camps.* Social Problems (1957-58) 5:230-243.

12660   SIEGEL, L. M.
Holocaust Survivors in Hasidic and Ultra-Orthodox Jewish Populations.
J Contemp Psychother (1980) 11:15-31.

12670   SIGAL, J. J.
Children and Social Catastrophe. Am Psychoanal Ass Annual Mtg,
Boston, 1968.

12680   SIGAL, J. J.
Second Generation Effects of Massive Psychic Trauma. In Krystal, H.
and G. Niederland (eds.), Psychic Traumatization. Boston: Little,
Brown, (1970) 55-65.

12690   SIGAL, J. J.; RAKOFF, V.
*Concentration Camp Survival. A Pilot Study of the Effects on the
Second Generation.* Can Psychiat Ass J (1971) 16:393-397.

12700   SIGAL, J. J.
*Hypotheses and Methodology in the Study of Families of the Holocaust
Survivors.* In Anthony, E. J. and C. Koupernik (eds.), The Child in His
Family: The Impact of Disease and Death. New York: Wiley, 1973,
43:320-327.

12710   SIGAL, J. J.; SILVER, D.; RAKOFF, V.; ELLIN, B.
Some Second Generation Effects of Survival of the Nazi Persecution.
Orthopsychiat (1973) 43(3):320-327.

12720   SIGAL, J. J.
*Effects of Paternal Exposure to Prolonged Stress on the Mental Health of
the Spouse and Children.* Can Psychiat Ass J (1976) 21:166-170.

12730   SIKORSKI, J.
[*Pharmaceutical and Sanitary Supplies and Facilities in the
Concentration Camps of Oswiecim-Brzezinka in 1940-1945*]. Arch Hist
Med (Wars) (1975) 38(3-4):283-298.

12740   SIMENAUER, E.
Late Psychic Sequelae of Man-Made Disasters. Int J Psycho-Anal (1968)
49:306-309.

12750   SIMENAUER, E.
A Double Helix: Some Determinants of Self-Perpetuation of Nazism.
Psychoanal Study of the Child (1978) 33:411-425.

12760   SIMENAUER, E.
Die Zweite Generation-Danach. Die Wiederkehr Der
Verfolgermentalität In Psychoanalysen. [*The Second Generation
Afterwards. The Return of the Mentality of Persecution in
Psychoanalyses*]. Jahrbuch der Psychoanalyse (1981) 12:8-17.

12770 SIMMEDINGER, A.N.
Neue Wege. Zur Bestimmung Verfolgungsbedingter Schäden An Körper Und Gesundheit Bei Naziopfern, Kriegsbeschädigten Und Sozialrentnern. [*New Approaches of Finding Disturbances Caused by Persecution in Nazi Victims, War-Disabled and Social Pensioners*]. In Michel, M. (ed.), Gesundheitsschäden Durch Verfolgung Und Gefangenschaft Und Ihre Spätfolgen. Frankfurt Am Main: Röderberg Verlag, 1955, 246–250.

12780 SINIECKI, B.
[*The Camp Hospital at Stutthof. An Outline of History*]. Przeglad Lekarski (1975) 32(1):85–89.

12790 SKOKNA, D.; KORHON, M.
Spätfolgen Der Tuberkulose Und Posttuberkulöser Pneumopathien Bei Mitgliedern Des ZPB/Verband Antifachistischer Widerstandskämpfer. [*Late Sequelae of Tuberculosis and Post-Tuberculosis in Members of the ZPB (Union of Antifascist Fighters)*]. VI Internationaler Medizinischer Kongress Der F.I.R., Prague, 1976.

12800 SKULIMOWSKI, M.M.
[*Ludwik Boleslaw Kotulski, M.D., (1888–1964)—Member of the Polish Underground, Inmate of the Pawiak Prison and Auschwitz Concentration Camp*]. Arch Hist Med (Wars) (1972) 35(1):181–184.

12810 SKULIMOWKSI, M.; SLIWINSKI, S.
[*Professor Wladyslaw Szumowski in Sachsenhausen*]. Przeglad Lekarski (1980) 37(1):144–146.

12820 SLIPP, S.
The Children of Survivors of Nazi Concentration Camps: A Pilot Study of the Transmission of Psychic Trauma. In Wolberg, L.R. and M.L. Aronson (eds.), Group Therapy. New York: Stratton International, 1978.

12830 SLISZ-ORYZYNSKA, M.
[*A Report from the Barrack No. 17 at the Women's Concentration Camp at Birkenau*]. Przeglad Lekarski (1978) 35(1):160–166.

12840 SOBCZYK, P.; CIELECKI, A.; ZEMBRZYCKA-CIELECKA, A.M.; KRUPKA-MATUSZCZYK, I.; KAZMIERCZAK, B.; LUKOSZEK, D.
[*Psychopathological Analysis of Preliminary Expert Testimony Materials with Regard to Former Prisoners of the Concentration Camps*]. Przeglad Lekarski (1980) 37(1):89–91.

12850 SOBOLEWICZ, T.
[*Experiences in the Auschwitz Hospital*]. Przeglad Lekarski (1984) 41(1):108–110.

12860 SOFLETEA, A.
Behandlung Und Weitere Prognose Des Erschöpfungs-Syndroms. [*Treatment and Late Prognosis of the Exhaustion Syndrome*]. In Die Behandlung Der Asthenie Und Der Vorzeitigen Vergreisung Bei

Ehemaligen Widerstanskämpfern Und KZ Häftlingen. III
Internationale Medizinische Konferenz. Liège: Verlag Der F.I.R.,
1961, 69–75.

12870   SOLKOFF, N.
Children of Survivors of the Nazi Holocaust: A Critical Review of the
Literature. Am J Orthopsychiat (1981) 51:29–42.

12880   SOLKOFF, N.
Survivors of the Holocaust: A Critical Review of the Literature. Catalog
of Selected Documents in Psychology (1982) 12(4):47. Ms 2507.

12890   SOLLADIE, R.
Klinische Und Biologische Ergebnisse Der Behandlung Von Folgen
Der Deportation Mittels Novokain Mit Niederem PH Wert Und
Zusätzlichen Medikamenten. [Clinical and Biological Outcomes of
Treating Deportation Sequelae with Low PH-Value Novocain and
Additional Drugs]. In Die Behandlung Der Asthenie Und Der
Vorzeitigen Vergreisung Bei Ehemaligen Widerstanskämpfern Und
KZ Häftlingen. III Internationale Medizinische Konferenz. Liège:
Verlag Der F.I.R., 1961, 2–26.

12900   SOMMERFELD, W.
Verfolgung-Gesundheit-Entschädigung.
[Persecution-Health-Restitution]. Referat Von Dr. Med Sommerfeld W
Gehalten Auf URO-Konferenz in Munchen (1961) 2–26. Manuscript.

12910   SONNENBERG, S.M.
A Special Form of Survivor Syndrome, Case Report. Psychoanal Q
(1972) 41:58–62.

12920   SONNENBERG, S.M.
Children of Survivors. Workshop Report. J Am Psychoanal Ass (1974)
22:200–204.

12930   SONNENBERG, S.M.
A Transcultural Observation of Post-Traumatic Stress Disorder. Hosp
Comm Psychiat (1982) 33(1):58–59.

12940   SPANJAARD, J.
Role of Self-Esteem in Concentration Camp Survivors. Tijdschr
Psychother (1979) 5(6):323–326.

12950   SPERLING, O.
The Interpretation of the Trauma as a Command. Psychoanal Q (1950).

12960   SPERO, M.H.
Psychophysiological Sequelae of Holocaust Trauma in a Jewish Child.
Am J of Psychoanal (1980) 40(1):53–66.

12970   SPRINGER, A.; BRATINI, E.
KZ-Haft Und Störungen Der Nachfolgegeneration, Eine
Untersuchung An In Ravensbrueck Inhaftiert Gewesenen Frauen Und
Ihren Kinder. [Concentration Camp Imprisonment and Disturbances in
the Second Generation. An Investigation of Female Ex-Prisoners from

the Concentration Camp Ravensbruck and Their Children].
Mitteilungen Der F.I.R. (1976) 10:26–29.

12980 STAEHR, H.
Neues Zum Neurose-Begriff Aus Der Sicht Des
Entschädigungsmediziners. [*Newer Remarks on the Concept of
Neurosis From the Viewpoint of Forensic Medicine*]. Deutsches
Generalkonsulat, New York, 1961. Manuscript.

12990 STASIAK, L.
[*Professor Robert Waitz. Reminiscences*]. Przeglad Lekarski (1979)
36(1):152–154.

13000 STEFANSKA, I.
[*Health Services at the Auschwitz-Birkenau Concentration Camp as
Pictured by the Inmates*]. Przeglad Lekarski (1977) 34(1):108–118.

13010 STEIN, J.; FENIGSTEIN, H.
Anatomie Pathologique de la Maladie de Famine. 1946. In Maladie de
Famine. Recherches Cliniques sur la Famine Executées dans le
Ghetto de Varsovie en 1942. [*Anatomical Pathology of Famine
Sickness*]. In Famine Sickness, Clinical Research on the Hunger
Deaths in the Warsaw Ghetto.

13020 STEINITZ, L.; SZONYI, D.M.
(Eds.). *Living After the Holocaust: Reflections by the Post-War
Generation in America*. New York: Bloch Publishing, 1976.

13030 STEINITZ, L.Y.
*Psycho-Social Effects of the Holocaust on Aging Survivors and Their
Families*. J Gerontol Soc Work (1982) 4(3–4) 145–152.

13040 STERBA, E.
The Effects of Persecution on Adolescents. In Krystal, H. (ed.), Massive
Psychic Trauma. New York: International Universities Press, 1968,
51–59.

13050 STERBOUL, J.
Therapie Und Diätik Der Verdauungskrankheiten Bei
Kriegsinvaliden, Deportierten Und Widerstandskämpfern. [*Therapy
and Diet in Diseases of the Digestive Organs of War Disabled, Deportees
and Resistance Fighters*]. In Fichez, L. (ed.), Andere Spätfolgen.
Austria: Verlag Der F.I.R. (1959), Band 2, 40–49.

13060 STERBOUL, J.; KRAWIECKI
Vergleichende Studien Der Dyspepsie Bei Ehemaligen KZ Häftlingen
Und Bei Greisen. [*Comparative Studies of Dyspepsia in
Ex-Concentration Camp Prisoners and in Old People*]. In Die
Behandlung Der Asthenie Und Der Vorzeitigen Vergreisung Bei
Ehemaligen Widerstanskämpfern Und KZ Häftlingen. III
Internationale Medizinische Konferenz. Luettich: Verlag Der F.I.R.,
1961, 127–135.

13070 STERKOWICZ, S.
[*Contribution to the Problem of Morals among the Prisoners in Nazi
Concentration Camps*]. Przeglad Lekarski (1969) 25(1):47–52.

13080   STERKOWICZ, S.
[*Pseudomedical Experiments at Neuengamme Concentration Camp*].
Przeglad Lekarski (1977) 34(1):130–137.

13090   STERKOWICZ, S.
[*Case of SS Physician Heinrich Schutz*]. Przeglad Lekarski (1977)
34(1):137–141.

13100   STERKOWICZ, S.
[*First Weeks Following the Liberation of the Neuengamme
Concentration Camp*]. Przeglad Lekarski (1978) 35(1):155–157.

13105   STERN, H.
Observations sur la Psychologie Collective dans les Camps des
"Personnes Déplacées" [*Psychological Observations in the Displaced
Persons Camp*]. Psyche (1948) 3:891–907.

13110   STERNALSKI, M.
Przyczynek Do Psychiatrycznych Aspektow TZW KZ-Syndromu. [*A
Contribution to the Psychiatric Aspects of the So-Called Concentration
Camp Syndrome*]. Przeglad Lekarski (1978) 35:25–27. Also in German:
Ein Beitrag Zu Den Psychiatrischen Aspekten Des Sogennanten
KZ-Syndroms. Mitteilungen Der F.I.R. (1978) 14:1–6.

13120   STERNBERG, T.
*Defence Mechanisms and the Working through of Resistance in Group
Therapy*. Group Analysis (1982) 15(3):261–277.

13130   STIERLIN, H.
The Parents' Nazi Past and the Dialogue between Generations. Fam
Process (1981) 20:391–394.

13140   STOKVIS, B.
Gedanken Eines Psychotherapeuten Über Das
Wiedergutmachungsverfahren. [*A Psychotherapist's Reflections on the
Problem of Restitution*]. Psyche (1962/63) 16:538–543.

13150   STRAKER, M.
The Survivor Syndrome: Theoretical and Therapeutic Dilemmas.
Psychiatry Digest, Laval Medical Canada (1971) 42:37–41.

13160   STRAUSS, H.
Besonderheiten Der Nichtpsychotischen Seelischen Stoerungen Bei
Opfern Der Nationalsozialistischen Verfolgung Und Ihre Bedeutung
Bei Der Begutachtung. [*Peculiarities of Non-Psychotic Psychic
Disturbances in Victims of Nazi-Persecution. Their Importance for
Compensation Decisions*]. Nervenarzt (1957) 28:344–350.

13165   STRAUSS, H.
Neuropsychiatric Disturbances after National-Socialist Persecution.
Proceedings of the Virchow Med Soc (1957) 16:95–104.

13170   STRAUSS, H.
Eine Partielle Entmannung. Seelische Impotenz Und Depressive
Lebenshemmung. [*A Partial Demasculation. Mental Impotence and*

Depressive Inhibition of Life]. In March, H. (ed.), Verfolgung Und Angst. Stuttgart: Ernst Klett Verlag, 1960, 60–66.

13180 STRAUSS, H.
Ein Entwurzelter Mensch. Eine Seelische Entwicklungs—Und Anpassungsstörung [*An Uprooted Person: Emotional Disturbances and Maladaptation*]. In March, H. (ed.), Verfolgung Und Angst. Stuttgart: Ernst Klett Verlag, 1960, 77–83.

13190 STRAUSS, H.
Ein Neunjähriges Kind Im Konzentrationslager. Enuresis Und Anpassungsstörungen. [*A Nine Years Old Child in the Concentration Camp: Enuresis and Maladaptation*]. In March, H. (ed.), Verfolgung Und Angst. Stuttgart: Ernst Klett Verlag, 1960, 77–83.

13200 STRAUSS, H.
Alle Freunde Verliessen Sie. Eine Angstneurose. [*All Friends Deserted Her. Anxiety Neurosis*]. In March, H. (ed.), Verfolgung Und Angst. Stuttgart: Ernst Klett Verlag, 1960, 67–76.

13210 STRAUSS, H.
Diskussionsbemerkungen Zu Vorstehenden Beiträgen. [*Discussion Remarks to the Preceeding Papers*]. Nervenarzt (1961) 32:551–552.

13220 STRAUSS, H.
Psychiatric Disturbances in Victims of Racial Persecution. Proceedings of III World Congress of Psychiatry, Montreal, 1961, 2:1207–1212.

13230 STRØM, A.
Purpose and Scope of the Examination. Study of a Group of Former Norwegian Deportees. In Later Effects of Imprisonment and Deportation International Conference Organized by the World Veterans Federation. The Hague: World Veterans Federation, 1961, 83–84.

13240 STRØM, A.
Undersokelse Av Norske Tidligere Konsentrasjonsleirfanger. [*Examinations of Norwegian Ex-Concentration Camp Prisoners*]. Tidsskr Norske Laegeforening (1961) 81:803–816.

13250 STRØM, A.; REFSUM, S.B.; EITINGER, L.; GRØNVIK, O.; LØNNUM, A.; ENGESET, A.; OSVIK, K.; ROGAN, B.
Examination of Norwegian Ex-Concentration Camp Prisoners. J Neuropsychiat (1962) 4:43–62.

13260 STRØM, A.
Norwegian Concentration Camp Survivors. Oslo: Universitetsforlaget; New York: Humanities Press, 1968. With papers by: Strøm, Eitinger, Askevold, Lønnum, Engeset, Løchen, Rogan, Haug.

13270 STRØM, A.
Method and Material. In Strøm, A. (ed.), Norwegian Concentration Camp Survivors. Oslo: Universitetsforlaget; New York: Humanities Press, 1968, 11–13.

13280   STRØM, A.
Time Prior to Arrest. In Strøm, A. (ed.), Norwegian Concentration
Camp Survivors. Oslo: Universitetsforlaget; New York: Humanities
Press, 1968, 14–17.

13290   STRØM, A.; EITINGER, L.
Arrest and Imprisonment. In Strøm, A. (ed.): Norwegian Concentration
Camp Survivors. Oslo: Universitetsforlaget; New York: Humanities
Press, 1968, 18–30.

13300   STRØM, A.
Work and Family Life after the War. In Strøm, A. (ed.): Norwegian
Concentration Camp Survivors. Oslo: Universitetsforlaget; New York:
Humanities Press, 1968, 31–35.

13310   STRØM, A.
Health after the War. In Strøm, A. (ed.). Norwegian Concentration
Camps Survivors. Oslo: Univesitetsforlaget; New York: Humanities
Press, 1968, 36–44.

13320   STRØM, A.; ROGAN, B.; HAUG, E.
Evaluations and Decisions. In Strøm, A. (ed.), Norwegian
Concentration Camp Survivors. Oslo: Universitetsforlaget; New York:
Humanities Press, 1968, 156–169.

13330   STRØM, A.
Krigsskader Og Krigspensjonering. [War Damages and War Pensions].
Lecture given in Bergen to Medical Association, 1970, Manuscript.

13340   STRZELECKA, I.
[The First Concentration Camp Hospital in Birkenau]. Przeglad
Lekarski (1984) 41(1):88–93.

13350   STRZELECKA, I.
[Development of Hospitals in Auschwitz-Birkenau]. Przeglad Lekarski
(1984) 41(1):84–88.

13360   SUAREZ, J.C.
Reflexiones Acerca de un Sobreviviente de los Campos de
Exterminio. [Some Reflections of a Survivor from a Concentration
Camp]. Revista De Psicoanalisis (1983) 40(1):35–55.

13370   SUSTA, A.; BARDFELD, R.; KANKOVA, D.
Zur Häuftigkeit und Dem Verlauf Bestimmter Rheumakrankheiten
Bei Widerstandskämpfern. [The Frequency and Development of Certain
Rheumatic Diseases in Resistance Fighters]. VI Internationaler
Medizinischer Kongress Der F.I.R., Prague, 1976.

13380   SUSULOWSKA, M.
Proba Interpretacji Tresci Snow Bylych Wiezniow Obozow
Koncentracyjnych. [The Interpretation of Dreams in Ex-Concentration
Camp Prisoners]. Przeglad Lekarski (1976) 33:13–17.

13390   SWAAN, De A.
The Survivor's Syndrome: Private Problems and Social Repression.
Israel-Netherlands Symposium on the Impact of Persecution. 2,

Dalfsen, Amsterdam, 14–18 April 1980. The Netherlands: Rijswijk, 1981, 85–94.

13400   SWAAN, De A.
Het concentratiekampsyndroom als sociaal probleem. [*The Concentration Camp Syndrome as a Social Problem*]. In de Swaan, A. De mens is de mens een zorg, opstellen 1971–1981. Amsterdam: Meulenhoff 1982, 140–150.

13410   SWAAN, De A.
De maatschappelijke verwerking van oorlogsverledens. [*The Social Working through of War Experiences*]. In Dane, J., Keerzijde van de bevrijding. Deventer: Van Loghum Slaterus 1984, 54–66.

13420   SYLLABA, J.
Flecktyphus In Der Kleinen Festung Theresienstadt, Böhmen. [*Typhus Exanthematicus in the "Little Fortress" in Theresienstadt (Terezin), Bohemia*]. VI Internationaler Medizinischer Kongress Der F.I.R., Prague, 1976.

13430   SYPIEWSKA, M.
[*Episodes from the Ravensbruck Camp*]. Przeglad Lekarski (1979) 36(1):175–179.

13440   SZCZERBOWSKI, K.
[*Reminiscences of the 1st Writer of the Auschwitz Concentration Camp*]. Przeglad Lekarski (1970) 26(1):198–201.

13450   SZUSZKIEWICZ, R.
Dentistry in the Auschwitz Concentration Camp. In Auschwitz, In Hell They Preserved Human Dignity, Anthology, Vol. 2, Part 1. Warsaw: International Auschwitz Committee, 1971, 184–197.

13470   SZWARC, H.
Chorowosc Bylych Wiezniow Hitlerowskich Wiezien I Obozow Koncentracyjnych. [*The Morbidity of Ex-Prisoners of Hitlerian Prisons and Concentration Camps*]. Przeglad Lekarski (1965) 21:38–46.

13480   SZWARC, H.
Krankheiten Ehemaliger Konzentrationslagerhäftlinge Auf Der Grundlage Der In Den Jahren 1964 Bis 1966 In Der Urpolen Durchgeführten Untersuchungen. [*Diseases among Concentration Camp Prisoners. Investigations Carried Out in the People's Republic of Poland 1964–1966*]. In Ermüdung Und Vorzeitiges Altern. Folge Von Extremebelastungen. V Internationaler Medizinischer Kongress Der F.I.R., Paris, 1970. Leipzig: Johann Ambrosius, 1973, 250–255.

13490   SZWARC, H.
Vorzeitige Alterung Der Ehemaligen Polnischen KZ Häftlinge Und Der Kombattanten. [*Premature Aging in Polish Ex-Concentration Camp Prisoners and Combatants*]. V Internationaler Medizinischer Kongress Der F.I.R., Prague, 1976, 1–2.

13500   SZWARC, H.
Über Die Betreuung Und Die Medizinische Rehabilitation Der Naziopfer Und Kombattanten. [*On the Treatment and Medical*

Rehabilitation of the Nazi Victims and Resistance Fighters]. In Cah d'inf méd soc jurid (1983) 19:150– 154.

13510   SZYMANSKI, T.; SZYMANSKA, D.; SNIEZKO, T.
The "Hospital" in the Family Camp for Gypsies in Auschwitz-Birkenau. In Auschwitz, In Hell They Preserved Human Dignity, Anthology, Vol. 2, Part 2. Warsaw: International Auschwitz Committee, 1971, 1– 45.

13520   SZYMUSIK, A.
Poobozowe Zaburzenia Psychiczne U Bylych Wiezniow Obozu Koncentracyjnego W Oswiecimiu. [*Postcamp Psychological Disturbance among Ex-Prisoners from the Concentration Camp Auschwitz*]. Polski Tygodnik Lekarski (1962) 17:86– 89.

13530   SZYMUSIK, A.
Post-Camp Asthenia Noticed with Former Prisoners of the Auschwitz Concentration Camp. In Auschwitz, It Did Not End in Forty-Five, Anthology, Vol. 3, Part 2. Warsaw: International Auschwitz Committee, 1972, 207– 240.

13540   SZYMUSIK, A.
Inwalidztwo Wojenne Bylych Weiezniow Obozow Koncentracyjnych. [*The War Disability of Ex-Concentration Camp Prisoners*]. Przeglad Lekarski (1974) 31:110– 112.

13550   SZYMUSIK, A.
Die Kriegsinvalidität Ehemaliger Konzentrationslagerhäftlinge. [*The War Disability of Ex-Concentration Camp Prisoners*]. Mitteilungen Der F.I.R. (1975) 9:10– 14.

13560   SZYMUSIK, A.; LESNIAK, R.; ORWID, M.; TEUTSCH, A.
Untersuchungen An Ehemaligen Häftlingen Der KZ-Lager Auschwitz-Birkenau, Durchgeführt An Der Psychiatrischen Klinik Der Medizinischen Akademie In Krakow (1959– 1976) [*Investigations of Ex-Prisoners of the Concentration Camps Auschwitz-Birkenau Carried Out at the Psychiatric Clinic of the Medical Academy of Cracow (1959–1976)*]. VI Internationaler Medizinischer Kongress Der F.I.R., Prague, 1976.

13570   TANAY, E.
Initiation of Psychotherapy with Survivors of Nazi Persecution. In Krystal, H. (ed.), Massive Psychic Trauma. New York: International Universities Press, 1968, 219– 233.

13580   TARGOWLA, R.
Sur une Forme du Syndrome Asthénique des Déportés et Prisoniers de la Guerre 1939– 1945. [*On a Type of Asthenic Syndrome in Deportees and Prisoners of War 1939–1945*]. Presse Médicale (1950) 58:728– 730.

13590   TARGOWLA, R.
Les Sequelles Pathologiques de la Déportation dans les Camps de Concentration Allemands pendant la Deuxième Guerre Mondiale.

[*The Pathological Sequelae of the Deportation to German Concentration Camps During World War II*]. Presse Médicale (1954) 62:611–613.

13600   TARGOWLA, R.
Bericht Zur Ausarbeitung Einer Neuen Rententabelle Für Ehemalige Verfolgte. Internierte Und Deportierte. [*Report about the Development of a New Pension-Table for Former Persecutees, Internees and Deportees*]. In Michel, M. (ed.), Gesundheitsschäden Durch Verfolgung Und Gefangenschaft Und Ihre Spätfolgen. Frankfurt Am Main: Röderberg Verlag, 1955, 274–280.

13610   TARGOWLA, R.
Die Neuropsychischen Folgen Der Deportation In Deutschen Konzentrationslagern. Syndrom Der Asthenie Der Deportierten. [*The Neuropsychological Sequelae of the Deportation to German Concentration Camps. The Syndrome of Asthenia in the Deportees*]. In Michel, M. (ed.), Gesundheitsschäden Durch Verfolgung Und Gefangenschaft Und Ihre Spätfolgen. Frankfurt Am Main: Röderberg Verlag, 1955, 30–40.

13620   TAS, J.
Psychische Stoornissen In Concentratie-Kampen En Bij Teruggekeerden. [*Psychological Disturbances among Inmates of Concentration Camps and Repatriates*]. Maandblad Geest Volksgezondheit (1946) 143–150. Also in: Psychiat Q (1951) 5:679–690.

13630   TAUBER, I. D.
Second-Generation Effects of the Nazi Holocaust: A Psychosocial Study of a Nonclinical Sample in North America. Ph.D. diss., Marquette University, 1980. Page 5210 in Vol 41/12-B of Dissertation Abstracts International. Order No: AAD81-10184.

13640   TAUFROVA, M.
Beziehungen Zwischen Der Psychischen Und Somatischen Seite Der TBC Erkrankung Im Konzentrationslager Ravensbrück Und Allgemeine Folgerungen, Die Heute Bei Der Einstellung Früherer Lagerhaeftlingen Zu Krankheiten Anwendbar Sind. [*Correlations Between the Psychic and Somatic Aspects of TBC in the Concentration Camp of Ravensbruck—General Consequences Applicable to the Attitude of Ex-Prisoners to Diseases*]. VI Internationaler Medizinischer Kongress Der F.I.R., Prague, 1976, 1–4.

13650   TAYLOR, B.
A Doctor against Hitler. Md State Med J (1975) 24(1):61–62.

13660   TENNANT, C.
Life Events and Psychological Morbidity: The Evidence from Prospective Studies. Psychol Med (1983) 13(3):483–486.

13670   TERRY, J.
The Damaging Effects of the "Survivor Syndrome." In Luel, S.A. and P. Marcus (eds.), Psychoanalytic Reflections on the Holocaust: Selected Essays. New York: Ktav Publishing House, 1984, 135–148.

13680   TEUTSCH, A.
Psychological Reactions during Psycho-physical Stress in the Cases of

100 *Former Prisoners of Auschwitz-Birkenau.* In Auschwitz, It Did Not
End in Forty-Five, Anthology, Vol. 3, Part 2. Warsaw: International
Auschwitz Committee, 1972, 143–173.

13690   TEUTSCH, A.; DOMINIK, M.
Neurosen Bei Nachkommen Ehemaliger KZ Lagerinsassen. [*Neuroses
in the Descendants of Ex-Concentration Camp Inmates*]. VI
Internationaler Medizinischer Kongress Der F.I.R., Prague, 1976,
74–78.

13700   THAYSEN, E. H.; THAYSEN, J. H.
Diseases of Deportation. In Helweg-Larsen, P. et al., Famine and
Disease in German Concentration Camps. Complications and
Sequels. Acta Psychiat Neurol Scand, Sup. 83. Copenhagen: Ejnar
Munksgaard, 1952, 71–80. Also in: Acta Medica Scand, Sup 274 to
Vol. 144.

13710   THAYSEN, E. H.; THAYSEN, J. H.
Medizinische Probleme Bei Früheren, In Deutsche
Konzentrationslager Deportierten. [*Medical Problems in Former
Concentration Camp Internees*]. In Michel, M. (ed.),
Gesundheitsschäden Durch Verfolgung Und Gefangenschaft Und Ihre
Spätfolgen. Frankfurt Am Main: Röderberg Verlag, 1955, 172–180.

13720   THOMPSON, L. J.
German Concentration Camps: Psychological Aspects of the Camps.
Inter-Allied Conf War Med (1942–45). (1947) 1:466–467.

13730   THOMSEN, S. O.
Eftersygdomme Hos Tidligere Koncentrationslejrfanger. [*Morbid
Sequelae Among Ex-Concentration Camp Prisoners*]. Ugeskrift For
Lager (1949) 111:665–668.

13740   THYGESEN, P.; KIELER, J.
Avitaminosis Incidental to Semistarvation. In Helweg-Larsen, P. et al.,
Famine Disease in German Concentration Camps. Complications and
Sequels. Acta Psychiat Neurol Scand, Sup 83. Copenhagen: Ejnar
Munksgaard, 1952, 207–234.

13750   THYGESEN, P.; KIELER, J.
Endocrine Glands. In Helweg-Larsen, P. et al., Famine Disease in
German Concentration Camps. Complications and Sequelae.
Copenhagen: Ejnar Munksgaard, 1952, 199–206.

13760   THYGESEN, P.; KIELER, J.
Mental Deterioration. In Helweg-Larsen, P. et al., Famine Disease in
German Concentration Camps. Complications and Sequels. Acta
Psychiat Neurol Scand, Sup 83. Copenhagen: Ejnar Munksgaard,
1952, 235–250. Also in: Acta Med Scand.

13770   THYGESEN, P.; KIELER, J.
The Mussulman. In Helweg-Larsen, P. et al., Famine Disease in
German Concentration Camps. Complications and Sequelae. Acta
Psychiat Neurol Scand, Sup 83. Copenhagen: Ejnar Munksgaard,
1952, 251–254.

13780 THYGESEN, P.
Allgemeines Über Die Spätfolgen. [*General Remarks on the Late Sequelae*]. In Michel, M. (ed.), Gesundheitsschäden Durch Verfolgung Und Gefangenschaft Und Ihre Spätfolgen. Frankfurt Am Main: Röderberg Verlag, 1955, 21– 29.

13790 THYGESEN, P.; FICHEZ, L. F.; LAROCHE, M.; JALOUSTRE, R.; SORNE, G.
Die Psychischen Symptome Der Heimkehr. [*The Psychological Symptoms of Homecoming*]. In Michel, M. (ed.), Gesundheitsschäden Durch Verfolgung Und Gefangenschaft Und Ihre Spätfolgen. Frankfurt Am Main: Röderberg Verlag, 1955, 52– 58.

13800 THYGESEN, P.; HERMANN, K.
Die Wirkungen Des KZ Syndroms, 19 Jahre Danach: Eine Medico-Soziale Analyse. [*The Influences of the Concentration Camp Syndrome 19 Years Later. A Medical Social Analysis*]. In Ätio-Pathogenese Und Therapie Der Erschöpfung Und Vorzeitigen Vergreisung. IV Internationaler Medizinischer Kongress Der F.I.R. Bucharest: Verlag Der F.I.R., 1964, 311– 326.

13820 THYGESEN, P.; HERMANN, K.; WILLANGER, R.
Concentration Camp Survivors in Denmark. Persecution, Disease, Disability, and Compensation. A Twenty-Three Year Follow-up. A Survey of the Long-Term Effects of Severe Environmental Stress. Dan Med Bull (1970) 22(1):78– 87.

13830 THYGESEN, P.; HERMANN, K.; WILLANGER, R.
Concentration Camp Survivors in Denmark. Persecution, Disease, Disability, Compensation. Dan Med Bull (1970) 17:65– 108.

13840 THYGESEN, P.; HERMANN, K.; WILLANGER, R.
Konzentrationslagerüberlebende In Dänemark. [*Concentration Camp Survivors in Denmark*]. In: Ermüdung Und Vorzeitiges Altern. Paris: F.I.R. 1970, 71– 125.

13850 THYGESEN, P.
Late Effects of Imprisonment in Concentration Camps During World War II. In Physical and Mental Consequences of Imprisonment and Torture. Lectures Presented at the Conference at Lysebu Near Oslo, 1973. London: Amnesty International, 1973, 69– 87.

13860 THYGESEN, P.
Notat Vedrorende Dodelighed Under Og Efter Deportation Til Tyske Koncentrationslejre. [*Note Concerning the Mortality during and after Deportation to German Concentration Camps*]. 1978. Manuscript.

13870 THYGESEN, P.
En Lovgivnings Intentioner Og Dens Virkninger. [*The Intentions of the Law and Its Consequences*]. Ugeskrift for Laeger (1979) 141:1164– 1169.

13880 THYGESEN, P.
The Concentration Camp Syndrome. Dan Med Bull (1980) 27(5):224– 228.

13890　TOL, Van, D.
KZ-syndroom, rampensyndroom en traumatische neurose.
[*Concentration Camp Syndrome, Disaster Syndrome and Traumatic Neurosis*]. I Medisch Magazine (1977) 16–22.

13900　TOL, Van, D.
KZ-syndroom, rampensyndroom en traumatische neurose.
[*Concentration Camp Syndrome, Disaster Syndrome and Traumatic Neurosis*]. II Medisch Magazine (1977) 62–71.

13910　TRACHTENBERG, M.; DAVIS, M.
Breaking Silence: Serving Children of Holocaust Survivors. J Jewish Communal Service (1978) 54:294–302.

13920　TRAUTMAN, E. C.
Psychiatrische Untersuchungen An Überlebenden Der Nationalsozialistischen Vernichtungslager 15 Jahre Nach Der Befreiung. [*Psychiatric Investigations of the Nazi Annihilation Camp Survivors 15 Years after Their Liberation*]. Nervenarzt (1961) 32:545–551.

13930　TRAUTMAN, E. C.
Psychiatric and Sociological Effects of Nazi Atrocities on Survivors of the Extermination Camps. J Am Ass Soc Psychiat, Special Publication (Sept–Dec 1961), 118–122.

13940　TRAUTMAN, E. C.
Fear and Panic in Nazi Concentration Camps: A Biosocial Evaluation of the Chronic Anxiety Syndrome. Int J Soc Psychiat (1964) 10(2):131–141.

13950　TRAUTMAN, E. C.
Violence and Victims in Nazi Concentration Camps and the Psycho-Pathology of the Survivors. Int Psychiat Clinics (1971) 8(1):115–33. Also in Krystal, H. and G. Niederland (eds.), Massive Traumatization. Boston: Little, Brown, 1970, 115–133.

13960　TREBING, G.
Blackfan-Diamond-Syndrom Als Folge Väterlicher Haftschäden [*The Blackfan-Diamond-Syndrome as a Result of Disturbances Caused by Persecution of the Father*]. In Ermüdung Und Vorzeitiges Altern. Folge Von Extremebelastungen. V Internationaler Medizinischer Kongress Der F.I.R., Paris, 1970. Leipzig: Johann Ambrosius, 1973, 255–259.

13970　TROSSMAN, B.
Adolescent Children of Concentration Camp Survivors. Can Psychiat Ass J (1968) 13:121–123.

13980　TSCHEBOTARJOW, D.
Wiederherstellungstherapie, Prophylaxe Und Behandlung Der Vorzeitigen Vergreisung Bei Ehemaligen Kriegsgefangenen Und Kriegsinvaliden In Der Sowjetunion. [*Rehabilitation, Prevention and Therapy of Premature Aging in Ex-Prisoners of War and War Invalids in the Soviet Union*]. In Die Behandlung Der Asthenie Und Der Vorzeitigen Vergreisung Bei Ehemaligen Widerstandskämpfern Und

KZ Häftlingen. III Internationale Medizinische Konferenz. Liège: Verlag Der F.I.R., 1961, 231–238.

13990 TUTEUR, W.
One Hundred Concentration Camp Survivors: Twenty Years Later. Isr Ann Psychiat Rel Dis (1966) 4(1):78–190.

14000 TYCHO, G.
Discussion of K. Hoppe, *The Emotional Reactions of Psychiatrists When Confronting Survivors of Persecution.* In Lindon, J. (ed.), Psychoanalytic Forum, Vol. 3. New York: Science House, 1969.

14010 TYNDEL, N.M.
Beitrag Zur Kasuistik Und Psycho-Pathologie Der Während Der Nationalsozialistischen Verfolgung Geborenen Kinder. [*A Casuistic Contribution to the Psychopathology of Children Born During the Time of Nazi Persecution*]. In Herberg, H.J. (ed.), Spätschäden Nach Extremebelastungen. II Internationalen Medizinische-Juristischen Konferenz in Düsseldorf, 1969. Herford: Nicolaische Verlagsbuchhandlung, 1971, 266–269.

14020 UTITZ, E.
Psychologie Zivota u Terezinskem Koncentracnim tabore. [*Psychology of Life in the Terezin Concentration Camp*]. Prague, 1947.

14030 VALKHOFF, J.
Psychiatrisering van politieke vluchtelingen en tweede generatie slachtoffers. [*Making Psychiatric Patients of Political Refugees and Second Generation Victims*]. Bull van de Klientenbond (1982) 10(4/5):26–29.

14040 VEEN, Van, A.
WUV-problemen, doktoraal skriptie over immateriele aspekten van de Wet Uitkeringen Vervolgingsslachtoffers 1940–1945. [*WUV-Problems (WUV = Dutch compensation law for persecuted). Thesis on Intangible Aspects of the WUV*]. Andragogisch Instituut R.U. Groningen, Groningen, 1977.

14050 VEGH, C.
Ich Habe Ihnen Nicht Auf Wiedersehn Gesagt. Gesprache Mit Kindern von Deportierten. [*I Did Not Get to Say Goodbye: Conversations with Children of the Deportees*]. Köln: Kiepenheuer and Witsch, 1981.

14060 VELLA, E.E.
Belsen: Medical Aspects of a World War II Concentration Camp. Paper 1. J R Army Med Corps (1984) 130(1):34–59.

14070 VENZLAFF, U.
Die Psychoreaktiven Störungen Nach Entschädigungspflichligen Ereignissen. [*Psychological Disturbances as Reactions to Traumatizations That Entitle to Restitution.*]. Berlin: Springer Verlag, 1958.

14080 VENZLAFF, U.
Grundsätzliche Betrachtungen Über Die Begutachtung

Erlebnisbedingter Seelischer Störungen Nach Rassischer Und Politischer Verfolgung. [*Principal Discussion on the Evaluation of Psychological Disturbances After Racial or Political Persecution*]. Rechtsprechung Zum Weidergutmachungsprecht (1959) 10:292–298.

14090   VENZLAFF, U.
Grundsätzliche Betrachtungen Über Die Begutachtung Erlebnisbedingter Seelischer Störungen Nach Rassischer Und Politischer Verfolgung. [*Principal Discussion on the Evaluation of Psychological Disturbances After Racial or Political Persecution*]. Mitteilungsblatt Der Notgemeinschaft (1960) 13:4.

14100   VENZLAFF, U.
Schizophrenie Und Verfolgung. [*Schizophrenia and Persecution*]. Neuen Juristischen Wochenschrift Beilage: Rechtsprechung Zum Widergutmachungsprecht (1961) 171–191.

14110   VENZLAFF, U.
Untersuchungen An Ehemaligen Norwegischen Konzentrationslagergefangenen. [*Investigations on Former Norwegian Concentration Camp Prisoners*]. RZW (1962) 7:295–296.

14120   VENZLAFF, U.
Erlebnisintergrund Und Dynamik Seelischer Verfolgungsschäden. [*Dynamics and Experiences in Psychic Disturbances Caused by Persecution*]. In Paul, H. and H.J. Herberg (eds.), Psychische Spätschäden Nach Politischer Verfolgung. Basel: S. Karger, 1963, 95–109.

14130   VENZLAFF, U.
Gutachten Zur Frage Des Zusammenwirkens Erlebnisreaktiver, Vegetativer Und Hormonaler Faktoren Bei Verfolgungsschaeden. [*Expert Statement on the Synergetic Action of Reactive, Vegetative and Hormonal Factors in Disturbances Caused by Persecution*]. In Paul, H. and H.J. Herberg (eds.), Psychische Spätschäden Nach Politischer Verfolgung. Basel: S. Karger, 1963, 111–124.

14140   VENZLAFF, U.
Mental Disorders Resulting from Racial Persecution outside of Concentration Camps. Int J Soc Psychiat (1964) 10:177–183.

14150   VENZLAFF, U.
Mental Disorders Resulting from Racial Persecution. Int J Psychoanal (1964) 45:617–621.

14160   VENZLAFF, U.
Über Die Ursachen Seelischer Dauerschäden Nach Psychomastischen Extremebelastungen. [*The Causes of Chronic Psychological Disturbances After Psychosomatic Stress*]. Proc Rudolf Virchow Med Soc (1964) 24:23–43.

14170   VENZLAFF, U.
Das Akute Und Das Chronische Belastungssyndrom (II). [*Acute and Chronic Stress Syndromes*]. Mediz Welt (1966) 17:369–376.

14180 VENZLAFF, U.
Die Begutachtung Psychischer Störungen Verfolgter. [*The Evaluation of Psychic Disturbances in Persecutees*]. Rechtsprechung Zum Wiedergutmachungsrecht (1966) 17:196–200.

14190 VENZLAFF, U.
Akute Und Chronische Psychiatrische Syndrome Nach Extremebelastungen. [*Acute and Chronic Syndromes after Extreme Stress*]. Med Klin (1967) 62:701–706.

14200 VENZLAFF, U.
Psychische Spätschäden Nach Gefangenschaft Und Verfolgung. [*Psychic Sequelae after Imprisonment and Persecution*]. In Herberg, H. J. (ed.), Die Beurteilung Von Gesundheitsschäden Nach Gefangenschaft Und Verfolgung. Internationalen Medizinische-Juristischen Symposiums in Köln, 1967. Herford: Nicolaische Verlagsbuchhandlung, 1967, 93–101.

14210 VENZLAFF, U.
Die Sachverständeigentaetigkeit In Der Wiedergutmachung. Bilanz Und Ausblick. [*The Specialists' Evaluations and the Problems of Compensation Status Today and in the Future*]. Rechtsprechung Zum Wiedergutmachungsprecht (1967) 18:594–595.

14220 VENZLAFF, U.
Erlebnisreaktiver Persönlichkeitswandel: Fiktion Oder Wirklichkeit? [*Personality Changes Caused by Life Experiences: Fact or Fiction?*]. Nervenarzt (1968) 39:539–542.

14230 VENZLAFF, U.
Forensic Psychiatry of Schizophrenia in Survivors. In Krystal, H. (ed.), Massive Psychic Trauma. New York: International Universities Press, 1968, 110–125.

14240 VENZLAFF, U.
Neuro-Psychiatrische Aspekte Der Voralterung KZ Überlebender. [*Neuro-psychiatric Aspects of Premature Aging in Concentration Camp Survivors*]. V Congrès Médical International F.I.R., Warsaw, 1968, 1–16. Also Manuscript.

14250 VENZLAFF, U.
Neurologische-Psychiatrische Ursachen Von Voralterung Und Frühinvalidität Nach Konzentrationslagerhaft Und Kriegsgefangenschaft. [*Neurological and Psychiatric Causes of Premature Aging and Incapacity in Prisoners in Concentration Camps and of War*]. In Herberg, H. J. (ed.), Spätschäden Nach Extremebelastungen. II Internationalen Medizinisch-Juristischen Konferenz in Düsseldorf (1969). Herford: Nicolaische Verlagsbuchhandlung, 1971, 82–89.

14260 VENZLAFF, U.
Neuropsychiatrische Aspekte Der Voralterung Konzentrationslagerüberlebender. [*Neuropsychiatric Aspects of*

Premature Aging in Concentration Camp Survivors]. In Ermüdung Und Vorzeitiges Altern. Folge Von Extremebelastungen. V Internationaler Medizinischer Kongress Der F.I.R., Paris, 1970. Leipzig: Johann Ambrosius, 1973, 259–265.

14270   VEYLON, R.
[*Camp Doctor*]. Nouv Presse Med (1976) 5(5):282.

14280   VIC-DUPONT; FICHEZ, L. F.; WEINSTEIN, S.
Die Tuberkulose Bei Den Deportierten. [*Tuberculosis in Deportees*]. In Michel, M. (ed.), Gesundheitsschäden Und Ihre Spätfolgen. Frankfurt Am Main: Röderberg Verlag, 1955, 91–100. Also in Fichez, L. F. (ed.), Andere Spätfolgen. Austria: Verlag Der F.I.R., Band 2, 77–88.

14290   VILLAR, H.; MIRANDA, R.
Efectos Alejados, Psicopatologicos, Medico-Legales y Sociales de las Persecuciones Raciales. [*Late, Psychopathological, Medico-Legal, and Social Effects of Racial Persecution*]. Rev Argent Neurol Psiquiat (1964) 1:289–297.

14300   VILLENEUVE, A.; DOGAN, K.
L'Adaptation au Milieu Contrôlé. [*Adaptation to a Controlled Milieu*]. Laval Méd (1971) 42(1):8–11.

14310   VISOTSKY, H. et al.
Coping Behaviour under Extreme Stress. Arch Gen Psychiat (1970) 5:423–448.

14320   VOETEN-ISRAEL, C.
Kinderen van oorlogsoverlevenden en hun voorgeschiedenis. [*Children of War Survivors and Their History*]. Thesis, St. Michielsgestel, 1982.

14330   VRIES, De, E. J.
Social Work in Connection with "Ways of Relating to the Traumatized-Persecuted." Israel-Netherlands Symposium on the Impact of Persecution. 2, Dalfsen, Amsterdam, 14–18 April 1980. The Netherlands: Rijswijk, 1981, 72–76.

14340   VRIES, De, E. J.
Relatie tussen de materiele en immateriele aspekten bij de hulpverlening aan oorlogsgetroffenen. [*Relation between the Material and Intangible Aspects in the Assistance to War Victims*]. ICODO-info 1 (1984) 1:6–15.

14350   WAITZ, R.
La Pathologie des Deportées. [*The Pathology of the Deportees*]. La Semaine des Hopitaux (1961) 37:1977–1984.

14360   WAITZ, R.; CIEPIELOWSKI, M.
Doswiadczalny Dur Wysypkowy W Obozie Koncentracyjnym W Buchenwealdzie. [*The Epidemic of Typhus Exanthematicus in the Concentration Camp of Buchenwald*]. In Piaty Zeszyt Poswiecony Zagadnieniom Lekarskim Okresu Kitleroskiej Okupacji. Przeglad Lekarski (1965) 21(1):68–69.

14370 WAITZ, R.; CIEPIELOWSKI, M.
Experimental Typhus in the Buchenwald Camp. In Auschwitz,
Inhuman Medicine, Anthology, Vol. 1, Part 2. Warsaw: International
Auschwitz Committee, 1971, 120–130.

14380 WAITZ, R.
*Pathological Changes Found with Former Women Prisoners of
Concentration Camps.* In: Auschwitz, It Did Not End in Forty-Five,
Anthology, Vol. 3, Part 2. Warsaw: International Auschwitz
Committee, 1972, 1–41.

14390 WAITZ, R.
Kind van de rekening, jeugdbelevenissen uit de Tweede Wereldoorlog
verteld aan Dick Walda. [*Children Who Have to Pay the Piper,
Experiences of Children from the Second World War Told to Dick
Walda*]. Odijk: Sjaloom, 1977.

14400 WALTER, F.K.
[*In the Shadow of Death. Reflections from the Sachsenhausen
Concentration Camp*]. Przeglad Lekarski (1977) 34(1):186–90.

14410 WANDERMAN, E.
*Children and Families of Holocaust Survivors: A Psychological
Overview.* In Steinitz, L. (ed.), Living after the Holocaust: Reflections
by the Post-War Generation in America. New York: Bloch, 1976,
115–123.

14420 WANDERMAN, E.
*Separation Problems, Depressive Experiences, and Conception of Parents
in Children of Concentration Camp Survivors.* Ph.D. diss., New York
University, 1977. Page 704 in Vol 41/02-B of Dissertation Abstracts
International. Order No: AAD80-17601.

14430 WANGH, M.
Psychoanalytische Betrachtungen Zur Dynamik Und Genese Des
Vorurteils, Des Antisemitismus Und Des Nazismus. [*Psychoanalytic
Views on the Dynamics and Recovery of Prejudice, Anti-Semitism and
Nazism*]. Psyche (1962) 16:273–284.

14440 WANGH, M.
*National Socialism and Genocide of the Jews: A Psychoanalytic Study
of a Historical Event.* Int J Psychoanal (1964) 45:386.

14450 WANGH, M.
Discussion to Hoppe in the Psychoanalytic Forum (1966) 1:75–85.
Psychoanal For (1966) 1:197–201.

14460 WANGH, M.
Forensic Psychiatry of Schizophrenia. In H. Krystal (ed.), Massive
Psychic Trauma. New York: International Universities Press, 1968.

14470 WANGH, M.
A Psychogenetic Factor in the Recurrence of War. Symposium on
Psychic Traumatization through Social Catastrophe. Int J Psychoanal
(1968) 49:319–323.

14480   WANGH, M.
Discussion of E. de Wind, Begegnung mit dem Tod. [*Encounter with Death*]. Psyche (1968) 22:447.

14490   WANGH, M.
Die Beurteilung Von Widergutmachungsansprüchen Der Als Kleinkinder Verfolgten. [*The Evaluation of Restitution Claims of Persecuted Children*]. In Herberg, H.J. (ed.), Spätschäden Nach Extremebelastungen. II Internationalen Medizinisch-Juristischen Konferenz in Düsseldorf, 1969. Herford: Nicolaische Verlagsbuchhandlung, 1971, 270–274.

14500   WANGH, M.
Verfolgungsbeschädigte Vor Deutschen Gutachtern. [*Persecution Casualties Facing German Restitution Experts*]. Psyche (1971) 9(25):716–719.

14510   WANGH, M.
On Obstacles to the Working through of the Nazi Holocaust Experience and on the Consequences of Failing To Do So. Isr J Psychiat Rel Sci (1983) 20(1–2):147–154.

14520   WANGH, M.
On Obstacles to the Working-Through of the Nazi Holocaust Experience and on the Consequences of Failing to do So. In Luel, S.A. and P. Marcus (eds.), Psychoanalytic Reflections on the Holocaust: Selected Essays. New York: Ktav Publishing House, 1984.

14530   WANSEM, VAN DER J.
Het verleden als het deel van het heden; oorzaken en gevolgen van stress in concentratiekampen. [*The Past as a Part of the Present, Causes and Results of Stress in Concentration Camps*]. Vrije Universiteit, Afd Klinische Psychologie, Amsterdam, 1979.

14540   WARNES, H.
The Traumatic Syndrome. Can Psychiat Ass J (1972) 17:391–395.

14550   WEBER, D.
Kritisches Zur Beurteilungspraxis Von Gesundheitsschäden Nach Verfolgung. [*Critical Remarks on the Evaluation of Health Damages after Persecution*]. In Herberg, H.J. (ed.), Die Beurteilung Von Gesundheitsschäden Nach Gefangenschaft Und Verfolgung. Internationalen Medizinisch-Juristischen Symposiums in Köln, 1967. Herford: Nicolaische Verlagsbuchhandlung, 1967, 52–56.

14560   WEINBERG, A.A.
A Comparative Mental Health Research of Jewish People. Isr Ann Psychiat Rel Disc (1964) 2:17.

14570   WEINFELD, M.; SIGAL, J.J.; EATON, W.W.
Long-Term Effects of the Holocaust on Selected Social Attitudes and Behaviors of Survivors: A Cautionary Note. Soc Forces (Int J of Soc Res) (1981) 60:1–19.

14580 WEISMAN, E. R.
The Rhetoric of Holocaust Survivors: A Dramatistic Perspective.
Dissertation Abstracts International (1980) 41(5-A) 1840.

14590 WELLERS, G.; WAITZ, R.
Effet de la Misère Psychologique Prolongée sur l'Organisme Humain.
[*Effect of Prolonged Psychological Stress on the Human Organism.* J
Psychol (Paris) (1947) 39:59–64.

14592 WERTHAM, F.
Looking at Potatoes from Below: Administrative Mass Killings. In A
Sign for Cain: An Exploration of Human Violence. London: Robert
Hale, 1968, 135–152.

14593 WERTHAM, F.
The Geranium in the Window: The "Euthanasia" Murders. In A Sign
for Cain—An Exploration of Human Violence. London: Robert Hale,
1968, 153–191.

14600 WESELUCHA, P.
[*Madness or Method? Post-Concentration Camp Reflections*]. Przeglad
Lekarski (1969) 25(1):181–183.

14610 WESELUCHA, P.
[*The Concentration Camp as an Experiment in Psychiatry*]. Przeglad
Lekarski (1970) 26(1):242–246.

14620 WETTERWALD, F.
Die Urologischen Spätfolgen Der Deportation Und Die Damit
Zusammenhängenden Rückwirkungen Des Vorzeitigen Alterns. [*The
Urological Sequelae of Deportation and Their Influence on Premature
Aging*]. In Fichez, L. (ed.), Andere Spätfolgen. Austria: Verlag Der
F.I.R., 1959, Band 2, 133–139.

14630 WIBAUT, F.
*Diseases and Disorders Resulting from Resistance Work and
Imprisonment.* In Later Effects of Imprisonment and Deportation.
International Conference Organized by the World Veterans
Federation. The Hague: World Veterans Federation, 1961, 126–145.

14640 WIELICZANSKI, H.
Observation on the Present Health of Former Nazi Prisoners. In:
"Poland" Illustrated Magazine. Warsaw, January, 1965, 19–20. Also
in Polish in: Przeglad Lekarski (1964) 21(11).

14650 WIESNER, N. A.
*Faith and Suffering: A Study of the Impact of Concentration Camp
Experiences on Moral and Religious Attitudes.* Ph.D. diss., New School
for Social Research, 1951. Page 3 in Vol W1951.

14660 WIJSENBEEK, H.
Is There a Hiding Syndrome? In Israel-Netherlands Symposium on the
Impact of Persecution, Jerusalem, 1977. The Netherlands: Rijswijk,
68–73.

14670 WIJSENBEEK, H.
Forty Years Later. Israel-Netherlands Symposium on the Impact of
Persecution. 2, Dalfsen, Amsterdam, 14–18 April 1980. The
Netherlands: Rijswijk, 1981, 66–69.

14680 WILDEN, H.
Die Entschädigung Wegen Schädens An Koerper Und Gesundheit
Nach Den Vorschriften des Bundesentschädigungsgesetzes (Beg).
[Restitution for Damages of Health According to the German
Restitution Law]. Nervenarzt (1963) 34:70–73.

14690 WILLANGER, R.
Eine Untersuchung Der Intellektuellen Reduktion Bei Ehemaligen
Deportierten. [An Examination of the Intellectual Decline in Former
Deportees]. In Ätio-Pathogenese Und Therapie Der Erschöpfung Und
Vorzeitigen Vergreisung. IV Internationaler Medizinischer Kongress
Der F.I.R. Bucharest: Verlag Der F.I.R., 1964, 327–333.

14700 WILLIAMS, M.; KESTENBERG, J.
Introduction and Discussion in Workshop on Children of Survivors.
Summarized in J Am Psychoanal Ass (1974) 22:200–204.

14710 WILSON, A.; FROMM, E.
Aftermath of the Concentration Camp: The Second Generation. Am
Acad Psychoanal (1982) 10(2):289–313.

14720 WILSON, D. M.
Note from New Zealand. In Later Effects of Imprisonment and
Deportation. International Conference Organized by the World
Veterans Federation. The Hague: World Veterans Federation, 1961,
148–149.

14730 WIND, de, E.
Eindstation—Auschwitz. [Final Destination—Auschwitz]. Amsterdam,
1946. (New edition, Amsterdam, 1981).

14740 WIND, de, E.
The Confrontation with Death. Int J Psycho-Anal (1968) 49:302–305.

14750 WIND, de, E.
The Confrontation with Death. Psychoanal Quart (1968)
37(2):322–324.

14760 WIND, de, E.
Begegnung Mit Dem Tod. [Encounter with Death]. Psyche (1968)
22:423–441.

14770 WIND, de, E.
Psychotherapy after Traumatization Caused by Persecution. In Krystal,
H. and G. Niederland (eds.), Massive Traumatization. Boston: Little,
Brown, 1971, 93–111.

14780 WIND, de, E.
Psychotherapy after Traumatization Caused by Persecution. Bull
Philadelphia Ass Psychoanal (1971) 21:3, 204–211.

14790 WIND, de, E.
Persecution, Aggression and Therapy. Int J Psychoanal (1972)
53:173–177.

14800 WIND, de, E.
Psychotherapy after Traumatization Caused by Persecution. Bull
Philadelphia Ass Psychoanal (1972) 22:1, 69.

14810 WIND, de, E.
Psychoanalytische behandeling van ernstig getraumatiseerden (door
vervolging en verzet). [*Psychoanalytic Treatment of Patients Severely
Traumatized in the Persecution and the Resistance*). Tijdschr
Psychother (1982) 8(3):143–155.

14820 WINKLER, G. E.
Neuropsychiatric Symptoms in Survivors of Concentration Camps. J
Soc Ther (1959) 5:4–11.

14830 WINKLER, G. E.
Probleme Der Psychiatrischen Begutachtung Der Opfter Der
Nationalsozialistischen Verfolgung. [*Problems of Psychiatric
Evaluation of Victims of National Socialist Persecution*]. Med Welt
(1961) 22:1226–1232.

14840 WINNICK, M.
(Ed.). *Hunger Disease.* Studies by the Jewish Physicians in the
Warsaw Ghetto. (Translated from Polish by Martha Osnos). New
York: Wiley, 1979.

14850 WINNICK, H. Z.
Holi Hanafesh Hameuhar (Ketotsa'ah Mipgi'ot Hashoah). [*The Late
Syndrome (due to Persecution)*]. Harefuah (1966) 5:175–278.

14860 WINNICK, H. Z.
Concentration Camp Survivors in Israel. In David, H. P. (ed.),
Migration, Mental Health and Community Services. Geneva:
American Joint Distribution Committee, 1966, 23–33.

14870 WINNICK, H. Z.
*Chairman, Psychiatric Disturbances of Holocaust "Shoa" Survivors of
a Symposium of the Israel Psychoanalytic Society.* Isr Ann Psychiat Rel
Dis (1967) 5:1, 91–100.

14880 WINNICK, H. Z.
*Further Comments Concerning Problems of Late Psychopathological
Effects of Nazi Persecution and Their Therapy.* Isr Ann Psychiat and
Rel Disc (1967) 5:1–16.

14890 WINNICK, H. Z.
*Contribution to Symposium on Psychic Traumatization Through Social
Catastrophe.* Int J Psycho-Anal (1968) 49(2–3):298–301.

14900 WINNICK, H. Z.
Psychological Problems after Severe Mental Stress. In Lopez, J. (ed.),

Proceedings, Fourth World Congress of Psychiatry, Madrid, 1966, Vol. 2. New York: Excerpta Medica Foundation, 1968.

14910   WINNICK, H. Z.
The Impact of Persecution. (General Background of the Problem in Israel). In Israel-Netherlands Symposium on the Impact of Persecution, Jerusalem, 1977. The Netherlands: Rijswijk, 1979, 18–24.

14920   WINNICK, H. Z.
On the Impact of Persecution. Introductory Remarks to the 2nd Netherland-Israel Symposium. Israel-Netherlands Symposium on the Impact of Persecution. 2, Dalfsen, Amsterdam, 14–18 April 1980. The Netherlands: Rijswijk, 1981, 9–14.

14930   WISHNY, S.
Children of the Holocaust and Their Relevancy to Probation: Presentence Investigation and Planning. Federal Probation (December 1980) 12–15.

14940   WITKOWSKI, J.
[*Dzierzana—A Branch of the Lodz Concentration Camp for Children*]. Przeglad Lekarski (1972) 29(1):151–157.

14950   WITKOWSKI, J.
[*Moringen—The Nazi Concentration Camp for Juveniles*]. Przeglad Lekarski (1972) 29(1):137–139.

14960   WITKOWSKI, J.
[*Sanitary Conditions Prevailing at the Myslowice Camp*]. Przeglad Lekarski (1975) 32(1):96–107.

14970   WITKOWSKI, J.
[*Sanitary Conditions Prevailing among Compulsory Labourers in "Festung Breslau"*]. Przeglad Lekarski (1979) 36(1):61–73.

14980   WITKOWSKI, J.
[*Juvenile Prisoners in Gross-Rosen*]. Przeglad Lekarski (1980) 37(1):118–128.

14990   WITTENBERG, C. K.
Children of Nazi Victims Seen as "Marked" by Stress. Psychiat News (1978) 34–38.

15000   WITTER, H.
Erlebnisbedingte Schädigung Durch Verfolgung. [*Damage due to Experience of Persecution*]. Nervenarzt (1962) 33:509–510.

15010   WITUSIK, W.; WITUSIK, R.
Slady Nastepstw Chorobowych Zwiazanych Z Pobytem W Wiezieniach I Obozach Koncentracyjnych. [*Pathological Sequelae Caused by Incarceration in Prisons and Concentration Camps*]. Przeglad Lekarski (1968) 25:56–64.

15020   WITUSIK, W.
Somatisch-Pathologische Veränderungen Des Sehorgans Bei Ehemaligen Konzentrationslagerhäftlingen. [*Somato-Pathological*

Changes of the Visual System in Former Prisoners of Concentration
Camps]. In Ermüdung Und Vorzeitigesd Altern. Folge Von
Extremebelastungen. V Internationaler Medizinischer Der F.I.R.,
Paris, 1970. Leipzig: Johann Ambrosius, 1973, 123–137.

15030 WITUSIK, W.; WITUSIK, R.
The Auschwitz Environment. In Auschwitz, Anthology, Vol. 3, Part 1.
Warsaw: International Auschwitz Committee, 1971, 105–151.

15040 WITUSIK, W.
Augenkrankheiten Bei Ehemaligen Konzentrationslagerhäftlingen.
[Diseases of the Eye in Former Prisoners of Concentration Camps]. In
VI Internationaler Medizinischer Kongress Der F.I.R., Prague, 1976.

15050 WLAZLOWSKI, Z.
[Hospital in the Concentration Camp in Gusen]. Przeglad Lekarski
(1967) 23(1):112–21.

15060 WLAZLOWSKI, Z.
[Pulmonary Tuberculosis and Treatment of Tuberculosis in the
Concentration Camp of Gusen]. Przeglad Lekarski (1968)
24(1):98–101.

15070 WLODARSKA, H.
[The Women's Hospital at the Brzezinka Concentration Camp].
Przeglad Lekarski (1970) 26(1):213–216.

15080 WOHLFAHRT, S.
KZ-Offrens Nuvarande Situation. [The Present Situation of
Concentration Camp Victims]. Svensk Laekartidn (1964)
61:4107–4124.

15090 WOHLFAHRT, S.
Aer Det Humant Att Tvinga KZ Offer Resa Till Vaesttyskyland Foer
Laekarundersoekning? [Is It Humane to Force Concentration Camp
Victims to Travel to West Germany for Medical Control?].
Laekartidningen (1966) 63:631–637.

15100 WOJTASIK, W.
Zmiany Chorobowe U Bylych Wiezniow Obozow Koncentracyjnych
Ze Srodowiska Kieleckiego. [Pathological Findings in the County of
Kielc (Poland)]. Przeglad Lekarski (1969) 25:18–24.

15110 WOJTASIK, W.
Zmiany Elektrokardiograficzne U 105 Bylych Wiezniow Obozow
Koncentracyjnych (Ze Srodowiska Kieleckiego). [Electrocardiographic
Findings in 105 Ex-Concentration Camp Prisoners (from the County of
Kielc)]. Przeglad Lekarski (1971) 28:10–12.

15120 WOJTASIK, W.
Zmiany Chorobowe U Bylych Wiezniow Obozow Koncentracyjnych
(Z Powiatow Wloszczowskiego I Staszowskiego W Kieleckiem).
[Pathological Findings in Ex-Concentration Camp Prisoners (from
Wloszczow and Staszow in the County of Kielc)]. Przeglad Lekarski
(1973) 30:21–29.

15130   WOJTASIK, W.
Najczestsze Zmiany Chorobowe W Ukladzie Krazenia U
Mieszkajacych Na Kieleczyznie Bylych Wiezniow Obozow
Hitlerowskich [*The Most Frequent Pathological Changes in the
Circulatory System of Former Hitler-Camps Prisoners, Living in the
Kielc Area*]. Przeglad Lekarski (1974) 31:75–82.

15140   WOJTASIK, W.
Nadcisnienie Tetnicze A Miazdzyca Uwagi Na Podstawie Badan
Bylych Wiezniow Obozow Hitlerowskich. [*Hypertonia and
Arteriosclerosis. Some Remarks on the Investigation of Ex-Prisoners in
the Hitlerian Concentration Camps*]. Przeglad Lekarski (1976)
33:80–84.

15150   WOJTASIK, W.
[*Arterial Hypertension and Arteriosclerosis. Remarks Based on
Examinations of Former Inmates of Concentration Camps*]. Przeglad
Lekarski (1979) 33(1):80–84.

15170   WOLFFHEIM, N.
Kinder Aus Konzentrationslagern; Mitteilungen Über Die
Nachwirkungen Des KZ Aufenthaltes Auf Kinder Und Jugendliche.
[*Children from Concentration Camps: Reports on the After-Effects of the
Stay in Concentration Camps in Children and Juveniles*]. Prax
Kinderpsychol (1958) 7:302–312.

15180   WOLFFHEIM, N.
Kinder Aus Konzentrationslagern; Mitteilungen Über Die
Nachwirkungen Des KZ-Aufenthaltes Auf Kinder Und Jugendliche.
[*Children from Concentration Camps Reports on the After-Effects of the
Stay in Concentration Camps in Children and Juveniles*]. Prax
Kinderpsychol (1959) 8:20–27.

15190   WOLKEN, O.
[*Liberation of the Oswiecimk-Brzezinka Concentration Camp*]. Przeglad
Lekarski (1966) 22(1):113–9.

15200   WOLKEN, O.
What I Think of Children. In Auschwitz, In Hell They Preserved
Human Dignity, Anthology, Vol. 2, Part 2. Warsaw: International
Auschwitz Committee, 1971, 13–20.

15210   WOKSKI, J.
[*Life at the Dachau Concentration Camp*]. Przeglad Lekarski (1978)
35(1):172–4.

15220   WORMS, R.
Rückfaelle Des Typhus Exanthematicus (Brillsche Krankheit) Bei
Ehemaligen Deportierten. [*Recurrence of Typhus in Former Deportees*].
In Michel, M. (ed.), Gesundheitsschäden Durch Verfolgung Und
Gefangenschaft Und Ihre Spätfolgen. Frankfurt Am Main: Röderberg
Verlag, 1955, 209–215. Also in Fichez, L. (ed.), Andere Spätfolgen.
Austria: Verlag Der F.I.R., Band 2, 161–169.

15230   WULFF, E.
Zur Frage Der Wesentlichen Mitverursachung Schizophrener

Psychosen Durch Verfolgungsbedingte Extremebelastungen. [*On the Problem of Essential Contribution to Schizophrenia Psychoses through Extreme Stress due to Persecution*]. VI Medizinischer Kongress Der F.I.R., Prague, 1976.

15240 ZABLOCKI, J.
W Rewirze Obozu W Sachsenhausen. [*In the Sick-Bay of Sachsenhausen Concentration Camp*]. Przeglad Lekarski (1977) 31:193–194.

15250 ZABLOCKI, J.
[*The Sick Bay at the Sachsenhausen Concentration Camp*]. Przeglad Lekarski (1977) 34:186–90.

15260 ZAGORSKA, E.
[*"Medical Review" Issues Dealing with Auschwitz*]. Przeglad Lekarski (1981) 38:224–229.

15270 ZASACKI, S.T.
Laborotorium Szpitala Obozu W Brzezince. [*The Laboratory at the Sick-Bay in Birkenau*]. Przeglad Lekarski (1978) 35:158–160.

15280 ZAWODZINSKA, C.
[*Reminiscences from Concentration Camps*]. Przeglad Lekarski (1974) 31:213–217.

15290 ZDAWSKI, T.
[*Preliminary Reports of Psychiatric Studies of Former Prisoners of Nazi Concentration Camps (Szczecin Area)*]. Przeglad Lekarski (1968) 24:64–65.

15300 ZELECHOWSKI, J.
[*The Dachau Concentration Camp and Its Hospital*] Przeglad Lekarski (1979) 36:163–164.

15310 ZIELINA, J.
Wynick Badan Lekarskich Bylych Wiezniow Hitlerowskich Wiezien I Obozow Konc. [*The Results of Medical Investigations of Ex-Concentration Camp Prisoners*]. Przeglad Lekarski (1966) 23:49–51.

15320 ZIELINA, J.
Block No. 9 of the Auschwitz I Camp Hospital. In Auschwitz, In Hell They Preserved Human Dignity, Anthology, Vol. 2, Part 1. Warsaw: International Auschwitz Committee, 1971, 198–208.

15330 ZLOTOGORSKI, Z.
Offspring of Concentration Camp Survivors: The Relationship of Perceptions of Family Cohesion and Adaptability to Levels of Ego Functioning. Compr Psychiatry (1983) 24(4):345–354.

15340 ZLOWID, W.
Stellungnahme Der Polnischen Organisation Der Widerstandskämpfer Und Opfer Des Naziterrors Zu Den Konferenzthemen Von Kopenhagen. [*The Attitude of the Polish Organizations of Resistance Fighters and Persecution Victims to the*

Themes of the Conference in Copenhagen]. In Michel, M. (ed.),
Gesundheitsschäden Durch Verfolgung Und Gefangenschaft Und Ihre
Spätfolgen. Frankfurt Am Main: Röderberg Verlag, 1955, 84–90.

15350   ZOBEL, J.
Zahnschäden Als Haftfolge. [*Tooth-Damages As Results of
Imprisonment*]. In Michel, M. (ed.), Gesundheitschäden Durch
Verfolgung Und Gefangenschaft Und Ihre Spätfolgen. Frankfurt Am
Main: Röderberg Verlag, 1955, 226–227.

15355   ZWERLING, I.
Psychiatric Studies of the Holocaust. Contemp Psychiat (1983)
2(2):134–138.

15360   ZWIERS-KLUVERS, I.; MEULEN-KLUVERS, VAN DER, E.
Is die oorlog dan nooit afgelopen? kinderen van ouderen met een
oorlogsverleden en met psychische problemen. [*Does That War Never
Stop? Children of Parents Who Experienced the War and Have
Psychological Problems*]. Avenue, mei 1978.

SUBJECT INDEX

The subject index serves as a guide to major topics of potential interest to the reader. It is a very rough guide indeed. For example, a number of articles are listed under *Effects* (general) and *Sequelae* for no other reason than the presence of these key words in the title. These articles could well be grouped together and also under such headings as medical, psychological, and psychiatric. Some of the articles refer to survivors; others to the children of survivors.

Articles referring to experimentation on camp inmates could be included as well with the *Medical Profession, Perpetrators, Camp Hospitals,* etc. The reader will simply have to review the seemingly related topics to sift out the relevant articles.

Where a reference number is bracketed, it does appear under one other heading. Where the title includes *Medical* and *Psychologic* effects, it deserves to be listed under the two main subjects. Psychological descriptions are to be found in the psychiatry section as well as vice versa, and the psychoanalytic articles could also be listed there.

The problems of creating a satisfactory subject index are considerable. Nevertheless, the editors hope that the following will expedite the researcher's search for relevant literature.

For those especially interested in the earlier literature, please refer to the Subject Index titled, The Early Literature, 1945–1960.

Adaptation and Coping
00470, 00570, 00730, (00750), 00760, (00790), 00880, 01940, 02590, 02600, 02610, 03650, 07070, 09540, 09620, 10170, 11660, (11800), (11970), (14310).

Aging, Premature Aging, Exhaustion, and Senility
02340, 02480, (02630), 03820, (03830), (03840), (03950), 04540, (05720), 08210, (08470), (08660), 09790, 10940, 12240, 12270, 12600, 12860, 13030, 13490, 13980, 14240, 14250, 14260, (14620).

Aggression
00520, (00580), (02000), 03320, (05470), 05640, (14790).

Arterial Disease and Arteriosclerosis
01010, 01040, (05720), 08860, (11160), 15140, 15150.

Asthenia
01290, (03830), (03840), (03950), 07170, 13530, 13580, 13610.

Cardiovascular and Cardiology
01510, 02850, 05040, (05080), 05160, 05800, 05810, (05820), 08340, 11590, 15110, 15130.

Children and Child Survivors
00680, 00890, 00970, 00980, 01260, 01970, (02160), 02950, 03510, 03960, (04130), (04290), 04570, (04800), (04980), 04990, 05110, 05120, 05445, 05450, 06300, 06310, 06470, 06490, 06500, 06850, 06860, 06880, 07030, 07080, (07200), 07240, 07730, 07860, 07870, 07880, 08000, 08220, 08230, 08320, 08480, 08450, (08550), 09150, 09390, 09780, 09940, 09990, 10020, 10021, 10560, 10870, 11200, 11210, 11220, 11680, 11700, 11870, 12180, 12190, 12710, 13040, 13190, 14010, 14390, (14490), 14940, 14950, 14980, 15160, 15170, 15180, 15200.

Cirrhosis and Liver Damage
01480, 02560, 02570.

Compensation, Restitution, and Pensions
00150, 00640, 01050, 01170, 01360, 01410, 01420, 01440, 01770, 01850, 02820, (03000), 03450, 03470, 03530, 03580, (03910), 05150, 05200, 05430, 05530, 05890, 06800, 06870, 06980, 07480, 07610, 07620, 08440, 08510, (08690), 08850, 08870, 08960, 08970, 09190, (09210), (09220), 09360, 09370, 09740, 09820, 09950, 10380, 11060, 11300, 11730, 12140, 12610, 12770, 12900, 13140, 13160, 13330, 13600, (13820), (13830), 13870, 14040, (14070), 14210, (14290), (14490), 14500, 14680, 14730.

Concentration Camp Syndrome and Survivor Syndrome
00230, 00480, (00510), 00550, (00560), 00670, 00810, 00820, 01085, 01740, 01750, 01760, 01780, 01790, 01930, 02160, 02260, 02280, 03030, 03060, 03070, 03230, (03400), 03540, 03550, 04240, 04430, (04810), 04820, (04850), 05140, 06340, 06400, 06520, 06950, 07160, 07500, (07690), 08730, 08940, 09840, 10140, 10350, 10360, 10410, 10420, 10550, (10570), 11320, 12090, 12100, 12910, 12930, 13110, 13150, 13390, 13400, 13670, 13880, (13890), 13900, 14540, 14850.

Concentration Camps (General)
00050, 00070, 00100, 00120, 00130, 00180, 00190, 00210, 00650, 00960, 01190, 01220, 01240, 01430, 01620, 01800, 01810, 01820, 02900, 02910, 02920, 03630, 03680, 04000, 04010, 04030, 04250, 04260, 04310, 04320, 04330, 04340, 04470, 04480, 04750, 04770, 04930, 04960, 05050, 05250, 05850, 05860, 05870, 05970, 05980, 05990, 06000, 06040, 06060, 06070, 06100, 06190, 06320, 06380, 6680,06690, 06710, 06720, 06930, 07490, 07800, 08120, 08270, 08630, 09050, 09310, (09430), 09570, 09630, 09680, 10030, 10280, 10590, 10600, 10770, 10990, 11000, 11010, 11020, 11100, 11120, 12020, 12310, 12380, 12450, 13100, 13430, 13440, (13720), 14020, (14060), 14300, 14400, 14600, (14610), (14960), (14970), 15030, 15190, 15210, 15280.

05370, 05380, 05420, 05650, 05790, 06140, 06240, 06920, 07520, 07530, 07540, 07580, 07780, 07930, 07990, 08030, 08050, 08260, 08330, 08520, 08550, 08710, 08820, 09090, 09130, 09530, 09670, 10400, 10460, 10680, 10810, 10830, 10950, 11180, 11410, 11790, 12170, (12250), (11260), 12420, 12950, 14190, (14310), (14590), 14890, 14910, 14920.

Famine, Hunger, and Debilitation
00410, 01840, 02370, 03140, 03660, 03860, 04120, 04400, (04510), 04620, 05060, 05070, (05080), 05090, 05230, 05680, (05820), 06910, (06990), 10740, 10750, 10800, 10840, 11150, (11160), (11530), 12050, 13010, 13700, 13740, 14840.

Family-Oriented Therapies
02290, 07830, 08300, 11960.

Genocide
00990, 01950, (02000), 03700, 09320, (14440).

Gerontology
00770, 00780, 01070, 01570, 01860, 02090, 02110, (05280), 05340, 06280, 06650, 08070, 09760, 10650.

Grief, Sorrow, Bereavement, and Mourning
00530, 00540, (00750), 01320, 06510, (07060), 09660, 09910, 12010, 12290.

Group Therapies
02070, (03970), (03980), (03990), 04050, (04130), (05220), 05940, 06960, (11280), (12200), (13120).

Guilt and Shame
01550, 01630, 04650, 11450, 11510, (12000), 12320.

Gynaecology, Amenorrhea, and Sexual Issues
04440, 04500, (04510), 04520, 04530, 06590, (06990), (07350), 07430, 09230, 10270, (11050), (14380).

Hiding
14140, 14660.

Individual Psychotherapy
(00580), 00610, 01670, 02770, 05490, 05500, 05510, 05560, 07650, 08310, 08880, (08890), 10250, (11980), 13570, 14770, 14800, (14810).

Medical Profession
(01330), (03710), 04780, 05840, (08790), 08800, 09380, (09430), 09830, 09900, 10620, 12460, 12470, (13090), 13650, 14592, 14593.

Medicine and Medical Problems
01000, 01020, (01030), 01060, 01200, 01210, 02010, 02180, 02330, 02640, 02660, 02670, 02880, 02890, 02960, (03240), 03490, 03500, 03770,

03870, 03880, (03910), 03940, 04680, 04840, 05010, (05170), 05180, 05190, 05260, 05310, 05320, 06560, 06620, 07210, 07290, 07300, 07390, 07410, 07420, 07550, 08130, 08530, (08660), 08910, (09240), 09440, 09450, 09460, 09470, 09480, 09490, 09500, 09520, 10180, 10490, 10700, 10710, 11520, 11750, 12350, 12370, (12400), 12440, 13050, 13060, 13480, (13540), (13550), 13710, (14060), 14110, 14620, 14640, 15100, 15120, 15260, 15310.

Music
08140, 08150, 08160, 08170.

Neurosis and Anxiety
00740, 01980, (02680), (02690), 02790, 03220, 05350, 06360, 09030, 09330, 09340, 09350, 09700, 10080, 11030, (11880), 12980, 13200, (13690), (13890), (13900), 13940.

Neurological Problems, Brain Damage, Encephalitis, and EEG Investigations
00240, 03570, 03580, 03590, (04280), (04290), 04300, 04700, 04710, 04720, 05920, 07180, 07190, (07200), 07220, 07750, 07760, 07770, 08930, 08950, 08980, 10110, 10980, (11530), 12620, 13760, 13770.

Ophthalmology
04910, 12390, 15020, 15040.

Parent-Child
(03960), 04040, 04380, (04970), 06790, 06810, (10200), 10210, 10220, (10610), (10760), 12680.

Perpetrators
(01180), (01330), 02550, 05330, 06090, 06160, 08180, (08790), (10620), (13090), (13130).

Personality Formation and Disorders
00280, 01080, 01500, 01910, (02990), 03340, 03890, 06010, 06030, 06050, 08580, (08700), 09100, (09210), 10820, 10850, 10860, 11330, 13070, 14220, (14930).

Physicians and Health Personnel in the Camps
01230, 01380, 03350, (03710), 04900, 07000, 07320, 07440, (07450), 07460, 07470, 07510, 07910, 08640, 08650, 08900, 09250, 09510, 10480, 10640, 11110, 11370, 11920, 12080, 12385, 12520, 12800, 12810, 12990, 14270.

Psychological Observations and Evaluations
00080, 00660, 00910, 00920, 01110, 01140, 01250, 01610, 01650, 01680, 01720, 01730, 02510, 02520, 03020, (03360), (04070), 04080, 04100, 04110, 04180, (04190), (04630), 04670, 04880, 05590, 05670, 05750, (06170), 06480, 06550, 06780, 07110, (07720), 07890, 07900, 08010, (08620), 08670, 08920, 09070, 09080, 09110, 09140, 09410, 09610, 09720, 09860, 09880, 09920, 09930, 10520,10880, 10890, 10900, 10910, 10920, 10930, 10970, 11310, 11380,

12070, 12210, (12400), 12500, 12510, 12840, 13105, 13520, (13540),
(13550), 13620, 13660, 13680, (13720), 13790, (14070), 14080, 14090,
(14160), 14180, 14550, 14690, 14900.

Psychoanalysis, Psychodynamics, and Defence Mechanisms
00870, 01110, 01310, (01340), 01690, 02450, (02760), 02780, 03010, 03440,
04640, (04730), (04740), 04760, (04800), 05480, 05520, 05550, (05940), 05950,
05960, (06730), (06750), (06760), (06770), 06820, 06830, 06840, 07630, 07700,
08020, 08060, 08080, 08370, (08380), (08680), 08760, 09010, (09150), 09170,
09180, 09400, 09650, 10010, (10200), 10300, 10370, 10390, 10790, 11440,
11490, 11500, 11830, 11850, 12120, 12280, (12360), (12760), (13120), 13360,
14120, 14430, (14440), 14510, 14780, (14810), 14870.

Psychosis and Schizophrenia
00350, 00360, 00370, 01890, 03110, 03170, 07660, 01260, 11550, (11790),
14100, 14230, 14460, 15230.

Psychiatry, Psychiatric Effects, and Psychopathology
00330, 01660, 02670, (02190), (02760), (02990), (03000), 03080, 03090, 03100,
03120, 03130, 03150, 03180, 03250, 03260, (03270), 03310, 03330, (03360),
03390, 03410, 03430, 03460, 03480, 03930, 04060, (04070), (04090), 04580,
04600, 06150, 06350, 07010, 07020, 07670, (07720), 08570, 08590, 08600,
08610, (08620), (08690), 09220, 09290, 09560, 09600, 09970, 10301, 10660,
10670, 11080, 11460, 11470, 11650, 13160, 13220, 13560, 13920, 13930, 13950,
14150, (14290), 14350, (14380), 14470, (14610), 14820, 14830, 15010, 15290.

Psychosomatic and Psychophysiological
00490, 00500, 00590, 01880, 03210, (3240), (03270), 04690, (04980), 05270,
05570, 05580, 05600, 05610, 05710, 05740, 05830, (08430), 10130, 10190,
10780, 11040, (11050), 11170, (12530), (12540), (12550), (12560), (12570),
(12580), 12960, (14160).

Pulmonary and Tuberculosis
02870, 03810, (03490), 05100, 05700, 06410, 07260, (07310), 10500, 10510,
12790, 13640, 14280, 15060.

Resistance Fighters
00380, 00900, (02630), 06180, (08390), (08400), (08410), (08420), (09240),
(10180), 10440, 10450, 12220, (13370), 14630, 15340.

Rheumatism and Arthritis
02490, 02500, 06260, 06270, (13370).

Second Generation
00110, 00160, 00200, 00250, 00260, 00400, 00420, 00430, 00440, 00450, 00460,
00800, 00830, 00840, 00850, 00860, 01100, 01120, (01340), 01350, 01400,
01490, 01870, 02080, (02130), 02210, 02250, 02460, 02470, (02680), (02690),
02700, (02730), 02750, 02970, 03380, 03600, 03610, 03620, 03920, (03970),
(03980), (03990), 04150, 04210, 04230, 04350, 04360, 04370, 04560,
04590,(04730), (04740), 04940, (04970), 05020, 05030, (05280), 05290, 05400,

05460, 06230, 06250, 06290, 06390, 06430, 06440, 06450, 06460, 06570, 06580, 06600, 06610, 06630, 06660, (06730), 06740, (06750), (06760), (06770), 06810, (06820), (06830), (06840), 06850, (06960), (07060), 07150, 07230, 07250, 07840, 07850, 08200, 08350, (08380), 08560, 08680, (08700), (08880), (08890), 09060, 09160, 09640, 10040, 10060, 10150, 10160, 10230, 10240, 10290, (10610), 10630, (10760), 11070, 11090, 11130, 11270, (11280), 11350, 11360, 11400, (11430), 11540, 11640, 11690, 11710, (11800), 11810, 11860, 11890, 11940, (11970), (11980), 11990, (12000), (12200), 12300, (12330), 12340, (12360), 12640, 12670, 12690, 12720, 12820, 12870, 12920, 12970, 13130, 13630, 13690, 13910, 13970, 14030, 14050, 14320, (14410), 14420, 14700, 14710, 14930, 14990, 15330, 15360.

Sequelae
00170, 00390, (01030), 01150, 01580, 01710, 02220, 02400, 02410, 02420, 02430, 03800, 04450, 04460, 04890, 05000, (05440), 05630, (06170), 06530, 06540, 06640, 06700, 07520, 07970, 07980, (08390), (08400), (08410), (08420), (08470), 09800, 09810, 09980, 10070, 10090, (10870), 11560, 11630, (12250), (12260), 12480, 12740, (12760), 13590, 13730, 13780, 14220.

Skeletal and Osteopathy
04200, 08280, 08990.

Suicide
01700, 11720, 12030, 12040.

Survivors and Survivor Families
01955, (04630), 04830, 05660, 05910, 06020, 07040, 07050, 07120, 07810, 07820, 07880, 08705, 08750, 08770, 08780, (08810), 08830, 09020, 09200, 09710, 09890, 10050, 10330, 10690, 11140, (11430), 11620, 11670, 11930, 11950, 12590, 12660, (12700), 12880, 12940, 13020, 13840, (14410), 14860.

Symptomless Interval, Latency Period, and Symptom Reactivation
00320, 02980, 05730, 09040.

Theoretical Issues and Terminology
01390, (07690), (07850), 10120, 10320, 10960, 11840, 12490, 12630, (12700), 12750.

Treatment and Rehabilitation
00251, (00510), 00600, 00620, 00630, 00710, 00940, 01090, 01160, 01470, 01830, 02050, 02060, (02130), (02190), 02270, 02380, 02390, 02580, 02720, 02860, 03190, 03200, 03790, (03830), (04390), 04660, (04810), 05300, (05440), 05690, 05760, 05880, 05930, 07650, 07710, 08290, 08500, (08810), (09540), 09690, 09750, 09850, 09960, 10100, 10530, (10570), 11340, 11760, 11770, 11780, 11820, 12160, 12890, 13410, 13500, 14330, 14340.

Typhus
00220, 00930, (01290), 02530, 02540, 03720, 03750, 03760, 07280, 13420, 14360, (14370), 15220.

The Early Literature, 1945–1960

00050, 00070, 00120, 00130, 00140, 00280, 00390, 00410, 00490, 00740, 00880, 00910, 00930, 00940, 01080, 01090, 01110, 01130, 01140, 01240, 01260, 01470,01510, 01590, 01700, 01720, 01850, 01970, 01980, 02330, 02360, 02370, 02380, 02490, 02530, 02790, 02830, 03840, 03010, 03030, 03040, 03660, 03680, 03690, 03700, 03720, 03790, 03800, 03810, 03930, 03960, 04050, 04060, 04130, 04170, 04180, 04190, 04390, 04400, 04410, 04570, 04580, 04620, 04690, 04750, 05040, 05060, 05070, 05080, 05090, 05100, 05230, 05240, 05250, 05310, 05320, 05350, 05440, 05680, 05700, 05750, 05770, 05840, 05870, 05920, 06150, 06240, 06300, 06310, 06360, 06470, 06900, 06910, 06990, 07140, 07520, 07600, 07610, 07660, 07670, 07750, 07760, 07770, 07780, 08480, 08930, 09070, 09330, 09340, 09350, 09360, 09370, 09750, 09800, 09810, 09820, 09870, 09880, 09900, 09980, 10280, 10300, 10520, 10530, 10800, 10810, 10820, 10830, 10840, 11030, 11050, 11460, 11520, 11530, 11560, 11570, 11580, 11590, 11600, 11730, 11740, 11750, 11910, 12130, 12240, 12400, 12440, 12650, 12770, 12950, 13010, 13160, 13165, 13170, 13180, 13190, 13200, 13580, 13590, 13600, 13610, 13620, 13700, 13710, 13720, 13730, 13740, 13750, 13760, 13770, 13780, 13790, 14020, 14070, 14080, 14090, 14280, 14590, 14620, 14650, 14730, 14820, 15170, 15180, 15220, 15340, 15350.

BOOKS

00070 ADELSBERGER, L.
Auschwitz, Ein Tatsachenbericht. [*Auschwitz, A Factual Account*].
Berlin: Letner, 1956.

00100 ADLER, H.G.; LANGBEIN, H.; LINGENS, E.
Auschwitz, Zeugnisse, und Berichte. [*Auschwitz, Testimony and
Report*]. Frankfurt: Europaische Verlagsanstalt, 1962.

00330 BAEYER, Von, W.R.; HAEFNER, H.; KISKER, K.P.
Psychiatrie Der Verfolgten. [*The Psychiatry of the Persecuted*]. Berlin:
Springer-Verlag, 1964.

00490 BASTIAANS, J.
Psychosomatische Gevolgen Van Onderdrukking En Verzet.
[*Psychosomatic Sequelae of Persecution and Resistance*]. Amsterdam:
Noord-Hollandsche Uitgevers Maatschappij, 1957.

00830 BERGMANN, M.S.; JUCOVY, M.E.
(Eds.) *Generations of the Holocaust*. New York: Basic Books, 1982.

00890 BERMAN, A.
*The Fate of Children in the Warsaw Ghetto in the Catastrophe of
European Jewry*. Eds. Y. Gutman and L. Rotkirchen. Jerusalem: Yad
Vashem, 1976.

00920 BETTELHEIM, B.
Surviving and Other Essays. New York: Knopf, 1979.

01140 BODER, D.P.
I Did Not Interview the Dead. Champaign: University of Illinois Press,
1949.

01720 COHEN, E.A.
Human Behavior in the Concentration Camp. New York: Universal
Library, 1953.

01810 COHEN, E.A.
The Abyss. A Confession. New York: W.W. Norton, 1973.

02020 DANE, J.
Keerzijde van de bevrijding, opstellen over de maatschappelijke,
psycho-sociale en medische aspekten van de problematiek van
oorlogsgetroffenen. [*The Reverse Side of the Liberation, Essays on the*

164   *The Psychological and Medical Effects of the Holocaust*

Social, Psycho-social and Medical Aspects of the Problems of War
Victims]. Deventer: Van Loghum Slaterus, 1984.

02420   DES-PRES, T.
The Survivor: An Anatomy of Life in the Death Camps. New York:
Oxford University Press, 1976.

02550   DICKS, H.V.
Licensed Mass Murder: A Socio-psychological Study of Some SS Killers.
New York: Basic Books, 1972.

02620   DIMSDALE, J.E.
Survivors, Victims and Perpetrators. Washington: Hemisphere
Publishing, 1980. With chapters by: Benner, Chodoff, Dimsdale,
Hamburg, Eitinger, Lifton, Luchterhand, Russell.

03130   EITINGER, L.
Concentration Camp Survivors in Norway and Israel. The Hague:
Martinus Nijhoff, 1972. First published by the Norwegian Research
Council for Science and Humanities, 1964.

03290   EITINGER, L.; STRØM, A.
Mortality and Morbidity after Excessive Stress. Oslo:
Universitaetsforlaget, Humanities Press, 1973.

03620   EPSTEIN, H.
*Children of the Holocaust: Conversations with Sons and Daughters of
Survivors.* New York: Putnam's, 1979.

03800   FICHEZ, L.F.
Andere Spätfolgen. Medizinische Konferenzen Der Internationalen
Federation Der Widerstandkämpfer Von Kopenhagen Und Miskau.
[*Other Late Sequelae*]. Austria: Verlag Der F.I.R., 1959, Band 2. With
papers by: Gukassian, Gilbert, Dreyfus, Franck, Sterboul, Heller,
Reicl, Worms, Desoille, Deveen, Wetterwald, Fichez, and Weinstein.

04060   FRANKL, V.E.
*From Death Camp to Existentialism, A Psychiatrist's Path to a New
Therapy.* Boston: Beacon Press, 1959.

04110   FRANKL, V.E.
Man's Search for Meaning. An Introduction to Logotherapy. Boston:
Beacon Press, 1962.

04600   GOTTSCHICK, J.
Psychiatrie Der Kriegsgefangenschaft. [*Psychiatry of Prisoners of
War*]. Stuttgart: Gustav Fischer Verlag, 1963.

04750   GRYGIER, T.
Oppression: A Study in Social and Criminal Psychology. New York:
Grove Press, 1954.

05190   HERBERG, H.J.
Die Beurteilung Von Gesundheitsschäden Nach Gefangenschaft Und
Verfolgung. Internationalen Medizinisch-Juristischen Symposiums in
Köln, 1967. [*The Evaluation of Health Damage After Internment and*

Persecution]. Herford: Nicolaische Verlagsbuchhandlung, 1967. With papers by Herberg, Ellenbogen, Lingens, Noordhoek-Hegt, Oyen, Linne, Venzlaff, Weber, Hoffman, Jacob, Brost, Paul, Paul-Mengelberg, Fischer, Dietze.

05210   HERBERG, H.J.
Spätschäden Nach Extremebelastungen. [*Late Damage After Extreme Stress*]. II Internationalen Medizinisch-Juristischen Konferenz, II Düsseldorf, 1969. Herford: Nicolaische Verlagsbuchhandlung, 1971. With papers by: Saller, Paul, Jacob, Schenk, Venzlaff, Klimkova, Amelünxen, Hoffman, Blaha, Lingens, Hackenbroch, Lønnum, Eitinger, Sheps, Paul-Mengelberg, Baeyer, Matussek, Klange, Dickhaut, Burgman, Lempp, Tyndel, Wangh, Hoff, Brym-Oyen, Ott.

06490   KEILSON, H.
Sequentielle Traumatisierung Bei Kindern. [*Sequential Traumatization in Children*]. Forum der Psychiatrie. Stuttgart: Ferdinand Enke Verlag, 1979.

07800   KRAUS, O.; KULKA, E.
Tovarna na Smrt, Dokument o Osvetimi [*Death Factory, A Document on Auschwitz*]. Praha, 1963.

07900   KREN, G.M.; RAPPOPORT, L.
The Holocaust and the Crisis of Human Behavior. New York, London: Holmes & Meier Publishers, 1980.

07990   KRYSTAL, H.
Massive Psychic Trauma. New York: International Universities Press, 1968. With chapters by: Bychowski, Danto, Hoppe, Klein, Krystal, Meerloo, Niederland, Petty, Sterba, Tanay, Venzlaff, Dorsey, Lifton, Souris.

08550   LEMPP, R.
Extremebelastung in Kindes-Und Jugendalter. [Über Psychosoziale Spatfolgen Nach Nationalsozialistischer Verfolgung in Kindes-Und Jugendalter Anhand Von Aktengutachten]. [*Extreme Stress in Children and Youth*]. Bern/Stuttgart/Wien: Hans Huber, 1979.

09170   LUEL, S.A.; MARCUS, P.
(Eds.). *Psychoanalytic Reflections on the Holocaust*. New York: Holocaust Awareness Institute, Center for Judaic Studies, University of Denver and Ktav Publishing House Inc., 1984.

09350   MARCH, H.
Verfolgung Und Angst. In Ihren Leib-Seelischen Auswirkungen. [*Persecution and Anxiety*]. Stuttgart: Ernst Klett Verlag, 1960. By Von Baeyer and Kisker, Cremerius, March, Strauss.

09380   MARCH, H.
(Ed.). Medizin und Menschlichkeit. [*Medicine and Humanity*]. Herford: Nicolaische Verlagsbuchhandlung, 1968.

09570   MATUSSEK, P.
Die Konzentrationslagerhaft Und Ihre Folgen. [*Internment in Concentration Camps and Its Consequences*]. Berlin: Springer-Verlag, 1971. Psychiatry Series. Part II. With: Grigat, Haibock, Halbach, Kemmler, Mantell, Triebel, Vardy, Wedel. English translation, 1975.

09810   MICHEL, M.
Gesundheitsschäden Durch Verfolgung Und Gefdangenschaft Und Ihre Spätfolgen. [*Disturbances of Health Caused by Persecution and Imprisonment and Their Late Sequels*]. Frankfurt Am Main: Roederberg Verlag, 1955. With papers by: Canivet, Deveen, Fog, Mogens, Hagen, Helweg, Hermann, Hoffmeyer, Kieler, Munke, Thaysen, Thygesen, Thaysen, Targowla, Dupont, Fichez, Gilbert-Dreyfus, Worms, Desoille, Richet, Blockhin, Reid.

09900   MITSCHERLICH, A.; MIELKE, F.
Doctors of Infamy. The Story of Nazi Medical Crimes. New York: Henry Schuman, 1949.

09910   MITSCHERLICH, A.; MITSCHERLICH, M.
The Inability to Mourn. New York: Grove Press, 1975.

10020   MOSKOVITZ, S.
Love Despite Hate. Child Survivors of the Holocaust and Their Adult Lives. New York: Schocken Books Inc., 1982.

10880   PAUL, H.A.; HERBERG, H.J.
Psychische Spätschäden Nach Politischer Verfolgung. [*Psychological Sequelae After Political Persecution*]. Basel: S. Karger, 1963. With papers by: Von Baeyer, Doering, Haenfer, Kluge, Mende, Bondy, Herberg, Fitzek, Kisker, Lingens, Paul, Mengelberg, Venzlaff.

10910   PAUL, H.A.; HERBERG, H.J.
Psychische Spätschäden Nach Politischer Verfolgung. [*Psychic Sequelae after Political Persecution*]. New York: Karger Verlag, 1967. 2nd Ed. With papers of the same authors as in the first edition and additional papers by Paul and Herberg.

12280   SCHIFFER, I.
The Trauma of Time. Analysis of a Concentration Camp Survivor. New York: International Universities Press, 1978.

13260   STRØM, A.
Norwegian Concentration Camp Survivors. Oslo: Universitetsforlaget, Humanities Press, 1968. With papers by Strøm, Eitinger, Askevold, Lønnum, Engeset, Løchen, Rogan, Haug.

14050   VEGH, C.
Ich Habe Ihnen Nicht Auf Wiedersehn Gesagt. Gesprache Mit Kindern von Deportierten. [*I Did Not Get to Say Goodbye — Conversations with Children of the Deportees*]. Koln: Kiepenheuer and Witsch, 1981.

14840   WINNICK, M.
(Ed.). *Hunger Disease.* Studies by the Jewish Physicians in the Warsaw Ghetto. (Translated from Polish by Martha Osnos). New York: Wiley, 1979.

THESES

00400, 00640, 00800, 01120, 01490, 01940, 02100, 02470, 03550, 03920, 04270, 04560, 04590, 04940, 04970, 06390, 07140, 07150, 07930, 07960, 08190, 08700, 09020, 09060, 09070, 09200, 09990, 10280, 10610, 10760, 11270, 11350, 11540, 11800, 11880, 11890, 12000, 12450, 12630, 12640, 13630, 14320, 14420, 14580, 14650.

THREE CENTRES WITH MAJOR COLLECTIONS

Those who use this bibliography may wish to obtain copies of certain articles. No one centre has all the literature listed.

The authors would be grateful if articles which may have been missed are sent to any of the three centres. A comprehensive collection exists at the University of Haifa and articles in Hebrew and available translations can be requested from there. Dutch titles are primarily located in Utrecht, whereas the North American literature is at all three locations. Each centre is completing its library to include *all* articles, whether in Polish or English, Hebrew or French. Requests and/or articles can be forwarded to:

HAIFA, Israel: Miriam Rieck, M.A.
                Ray D. Wolfe Centre for Study of Psychological Stress,
                University of Haifa,
                Mount Carmel,
                Haifa, Israel
UTRECHT, Holland:
                Nick Vos, Ph.D.
                Stichting ICODO,
                Willem Barentszstraat 31C,
                3572 PB Utrecht,
                The Netherlands
VANCOUVER, Canada:
                Robert Krell, M.D.
                Department of Psychiatry,
                Health Sciences Centre Hospital,
                University of British Columbia,
                Vancouver, B.C. V6T 2A1